Evidence-Based Nursing Care for Stroke and Neurovascular Conditions

Editor

Sheila A. Alexander, RN, PhD
Assistant Professor
Acute and Tertiary Care
School of Nursing
University of Pittsburgh
Pittsburgh, PA, USA

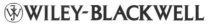

A John Wiley & Sons, Inc., Publication

Editorial offices   2121 State Avenue, Ames, Iowa 50014-8300, USA
               The Atrium, Southern Gate, Chichester, West Sussex, PO19 8SQ, UK
               9600 Garsington Road, Oxford, OX4 2DQ, UK

For details of our global editorial offices, for customer services and for information about how to apply for permission to reuse the copyright material in this book please see our website at www.wiley.com/wiley-blackwell.

Library of Congress Cataloging-in-Publication Data
Evidence-based nursing care for stroke and neurovascular conditions / editor
Sheila A. Alexander.
    p. cm.
  Includes bibliographical references and index.
  ISBN 978-0-470-95875-9 (pbk. : alk. paper)   1. Cerebrovascular disease–Treatment.
2. Evidence-based nursing.   I. Alexander, Sheila A.
  RC388.5.E976 2013
  616.8'10231–dc23

                                                              2012028347

A catalogue record for this book is available from the British Library.

"Nursing encompasses an art, a humanistic orientation, a feeling for the value of the individual, and an intuitive sense of ethics, and of the appropriateness of action taken."

Myrtle Aydelotte, PhD, RN, FAAN

Contents

Contents

Contributors

Tarek Dakakni, MD
Translational Acute Brain Injury Research Group
Department of Anesthesiology
Department of Medicine (Neurology)
Duke University
Durham, North Carolina, USA

Alice E. Davis, PhD, APRN
Assistant Professor
School of Nursing
University of Hawaii, Hilo
Hilo, Hawaii, USA

Michael L. "Luke" James, MD
Assistant Professor
Translational Acute Brain Injury Research Group
Department of Anesthesiology
Department of Medicine (Neurology)
Duke University
Durham, North Carolina, USA

Lori M. Massaro, MSN, CRNP
Clinical Supervisor
UPMC Stroke Institute
Pittsburgh, Pennsylvania, USA

Preface

Nursing is a profession that requires significant didactic and clinical training for entry into practice. Development into an expert in this field, as with any other, requires scholarly inquiry, continuous evaluation of current practices, and experience only gained over time. There are limited resources available for the neuroscience nurse, and even fewer specific to those who further specialize in the neurovascular nursing specialty. An aging population has been supported by advancements in care allowing individuals to survive who once would not, and an increase in population growth have led to a larger aging population with significant neurovascular disease. These changes have led to an increase in both quantity and quality of life, but also an increase in workload for health care providers and a need for knowledge about the evidence driving care practices including diagnostic tools and surgical, medical, and behavioral interventions. Nursing, neuroscience nursing, and neurovascular nursing in particular are advancing at a rapid pace. Increased knowledge about pathology driving various diseases has led to rapid advancements in care including newly developed interventions and challenges to existing treatment protocols that are known to lack efficacy. It is difficult for the new bedside nurse and for the practicing nurse to develop and maintain expertise within the context of rapidly changing standard of care protocols. Patients are better served by clinicians with specialized knowledge and experience in similar populations. As we continue to focus on more specialized areas of care and populations, it becomes more and more difficult for the clinician at any point in the spectrum to keep up on best practices to maximize patient outcomes. There are few text resources for the neuroscience nurse, and while there are some very excellent texts available, there are none specific to neurovascular nursing. The complexity of neurovascular disease and the body's response to critical events in the context of pre-existing co-morbidities requires nurses to provide care based on evidence, but also perform critical thinking that requires a strong knowledge base and foundation for care. The special needs of these patients' demands that nurses have detailed knowledge of the pathophysiologic underpinnings driving disease development, progression, symptoms, and the care we provide. This book was written out of the need for bedside nurses from novice to expert in all roles for a single source to begin the learning process around the area of neurovascular nursing. It is meant to serve the novice nurse as a single source to initiate the process of development into expert, but also to serve the expert nurse as a source of reference for existing care and foundational understanding to aid in the development of standard protocols. It brings together the knowledge gained through personal experiences of the various contributors, a lifetime of mentors, and an exhaustive search of the literature to find rationale for current practices.

This book is the first effort to bring together knowledge from the many disciplines on which nursing draws to develop a framework for care of some common and not so common neurovascular diseases. Each chapter includes a clear description of the known pathophysiology of the disease process and the impact that pathophysiology has on individual patients. Current evidence-based care is described with rationale for each intervention provided. In cases where there is no proven, efficacious treatment regimen available, a current state of the knowledge of existing treatments with appropriate rationale has been provided. This has been provided to promote the understanding of disease and interventions and critical thinking. It is not meant to be the final decision for patient care, but rather a starting point upon which nurses can gain meaningful command of the knowledge and build on that understanding to offer individual patients the best care. It has also been written so that the reader may better understand the impact of as yet unidentified interventions and their potential impact on patient recovery.

Acknowledgments

There has been considerable effort on the part of many individuals resulting in this final book. I would like to extend appreciation and thanks to each of those people because without their input this final product would never have been completed. My colleague and friend, Gretchen Zewe, worked with me to identify the most clinically necessary topics for this book and identify others with appropriate expertise to assist in the writing. The other contributing authors of this book, Lori M. Massaro, Alice E. Davis, Tarek Dakakni, and (Michael) Luke James have my eternal gratitude for thankless sharing of their time, energy, experience, expertise, and brain power to produce this work. Additional recognition and thanks go out to Melissa Wahl, Senior Editorial Assistant, and Carrie Horn, Senior Production Editor, at Wiley for their pleasant and persistent tolerance of my untraditional working style. Finally to my colleagues, friends, family, and my dear husband who were so supportive as I worked on this piece. It is through the efforts of all of these individuals that this final product has come to fruition.

Evidence-Based Nursing Care for Stroke and Neurovascular Conditions

Introduction

1

Sheila A. Alexander

Evidence-Based Nursing Care for Stroke and Neurovascular Conditions,
First Edition. Edited by Sheila A. Alexander.
© 2013 John Wiley & Sons, Inc. Published 2013 by John Wiley & Sons, Inc.

NEUROVASCULAR NURSING

With the advancement of health care, several subspecialties have developed within the discipline of nursing. Neuroscience nursing was one of the first specialties, with the American Association of Neuroscience Nursing being established in 1968. The complexity of the central nervous system (CNS), disease processes impacting the CNS, and further advancements in health care of this population has resulted in increased specialization within neuroscience nursing. Neuroscience nurses now practice in clinical settings that specialize in spinal cord injury, traumatic brain injury, neuro-oncology, medical neurology, surgical neurology, neurovascular conditions, neurologic rehabilitation (some of which have specialty units within the overall setting), and general medical practices. They provide neuroscience specific care, as well as general care, to patients in inpatient settings, outpatient settings, community settings, and in individual's homes. The neurologic specialized educational needs of these nurses are vast, and available resources for nurses practicing in these settings are scarce. This book will serve as a resource for nurses providing care at all levels to individuals suffering from neurovascular conditions.

SPECIALIZED CELLS OF THE CENTRAL NERVOUS SYSTEM
Neurons

Neurons are specialized cells that reside within the CNS, and some extend out to organs and tissues within the body making up the peripheral nervous system. The structure of neurons is variable, with some common features (Figure 1.1). The dendrites of the neuron serve to receive chemical signals from other neurons. The soma, or cell body, of the neuron houses the nucleus and many organelles. Transcription and translation, resulting in protein production, occurs in the soma. The axon of the neuron carries the chemical signal from the dendrites/soma to the axon terminal, often called the buton. There are many microfilaments and microtubules within the axon that serve to maintain form and as a tract for transportation of substances made in the soma to the axon terminal. The structures of the neuron are important for neuronal communication. In a resting state, the extracellular fluid is more positive than the intracellular fluid. When a signal is received by the dendrite, the cell membrane becomes depolarized and positive ions flow into

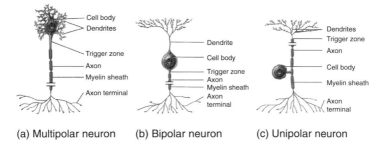

(a) Multipolar neuron   (b) Bipolar neuron   (c) Unipolar neuron

Fig. 1.1 Structural classification of neurons showing dendrite(s), soma, and axon. Breaks indicate that axons are longer than shown. Reprinted from Tortora, G. J. and Derrickson, B. (2009). *Principles of anatomy and physiology*. Hoboken, NJ: John Wiley & Sons, Inc. with permission.

the cell so that the intracellular fluid is more positive than the extracellular fluid. This is known as the **depolarization** phase of the action potential. Upon reaching maximum membrane polarization, ion channels close so no further ion influx occurs, and sodium-potassium pumps are activated to pump sodium ions out of the cell in exchange for fewer potassium ions. These pumps serve to restore homeostasis within the cell, bringing the membrane polarization to its normal range. The polarization normalizes during the **repolarization** phase of an action potential. As there is some delay in cellular recognition of the membrane polarization returning to normal, the polarization drops below normal so that the intracellular fluid is more negative than normal and then rises to normal again. This is known as the **hyperpolarization** phase. When the action potential reaches the end of the neuron, and the axon terminal depolarizes, vesicles filled with neurotransmitters move to the edge of the cell membrane, merging with that membrane and dumping their contents out of the neuron and into the synaptic cleft (see Figure 1.2). The neurotransmitter released will bind with receptors on the cell upon which the original neuron synapsed and generate action within the receiving neuron. Some neurotransmitters are excitatory, initiating an action potential in the receiving cell. Other neurotransmitters are inhibitory, blocking an action potential being passed on to the receiving cell. It is through a balance of excitatory

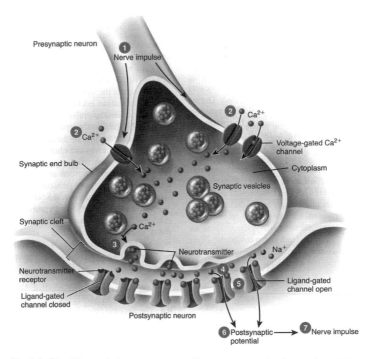

Fig. 1.2 Signal transmission at a synapse. Through exocytosis of synaptic vesicles, a presynaptic neuron releases neurotransmitter molecules. After diffusing across the synaptic cleft, the neurotransmitter binds to receptors in the plasma membrane of the postsynaptic neuron and produces a postsynaptic potential. Reprinted from Tortora, G. J. and Derrickson, B. (2009). *Principles of anatomy and physiology*. Hoboken, NJ: John Wiley & Sons, Inc. with permission.

and inhibitory communications that neurons drive functions within the body.

Neurons also communicate with cells outside the central nervous system. Neurons of the peripheral nervous system synapse on organs or muscle cells. When the neurotransmitters are released onto the cells of organs or muscles, they generate an additional response of that organ or muscle. For instance, peripheral nervous system neurons synapse on muscle cells in the thigh. These neurons release acetylcholine, which binds with nicotinic acetylcholine receptors on the muscle cell. Receptor binding causes calcium release within the cell and muscle cell contraction. In this way, neuronal input controls movement of the thigh. The movement of the muscle is modified by input from sensory neurons, neurons within the cerebellum, basal ganglia, and other brain structures to provide coordinated smooth movement.

It is important to note that there is structural variability of neurons within the CNS. Many neurons have a series of dendrites branching off the soma and one axon; this is the simplest neuron cell structure. Some neurons within the CNS also develop axons that branch into two axons that synapse on different cells, permitting one neuron to communicate with more than one cell (Figure 1.1). The axon terminals of neurons often have several branches so that one neuron can stimulate many other cells. This structure permits complex communication among cells that coordinate movement, maintain homeostasis of the body, and permit thought.

Astrocytes

While the neurons are the most widely known cells of the CNS, astrocytes are a vital cell type to CNS function. They are star shaped in structure (Figure 1.3a). In the developing brain, astrocytes release factors that stimulate stem cell differentiation into neurons. Astrocytes contribute to the blood brain barrier by extending portions of their cellular membrane, known as astrocytic feet, to wrap around the microvasculature and regulating substances passing from the blood into the CNS (Figure 1.3b). They stimulate transportation of nutrients, such as glucose and lactate, from the blood into the CNS and to neurons. Astrocytes absorb potassium from the extracellular environment, maintaining a proper environment to maximize neuronal function. They remove excess neurotransmitter from the synaptic cleft. Astrocytes are also able to release select neurotransmitters in select situations. When stimulated by neuronal release of ATP, they stimulate myelin formation by oligodendrocytes. Astrocytes can also become phagocytic, engulfing and digesting injured cells of the CNS, filling the space created by loss of these cells, and ultimately repairing/replacing the lost cells (Figure 1.3).

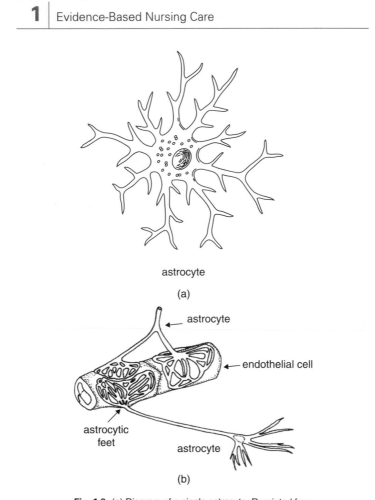

astrocyte

(a)

astrocyte

endothelial cell

astrocytic
feet

astrocyte

(b)

Fig. 1.3 (a) Diagram of a single astrocyte. Reprinted from Abbott, N. J. (2002). (b) Astrocytes and endothelial cells of the blood brain barrier. *Journal of Anatomy*, 200: 629–638. doi: 10.1046/j.1469-7580.2002.00064.x with permission from John Wiley & Sons, Inc.

Microglia

The blood brain barrier serves to control passage of many substances and cells from the blood into the CNS. While it serves to prevent CNS infection, once infection develops in the CNS, inflammatory and immune cells are not able to pass through the blood brain barrier to fight off infection. Microglia serve as macrophages of the CNS, scavenging for damaged cells, plaques, and infectious agents. Some microglia are phagocytic, engulfing and digesting their target. Once they have phagocytosed an infectious agent, they are able to act as antigen-presenting cells. Microglia can also release cytokines and other modifiers of inflammation. Many microglia lay dormant within the CNS and are activated when there is CNS damage or infection (Figure 1.4).

Oligodendrocytes

Oligodendrocytes serve to generate myelin. Processes of the oligodendrocyte extend out and wrap around the axon of a neuron. The oligodendrocyte cell membrane forms the myelin sheath. Myelin is wrapped around axons and prevents dissipation of action potentials by decreasing ion leakage out of the axon. Myelination of an axon permits the action potential to be transferred down the axon at its original strength over a shorter period of time. A single oligodendrocyte may branch multiple processes wrapping around the same neuron. Multiple oligodendrocytes may extend myelin sheath around the same axon. The gaps causes between myelin sheaths are known as the Nodes of Ranvier. Schwann cells are oligodendrocytes present in the peripheral nervous system (Figure 1.5).

BRAIN STRUCTURE

The brain is made up of multiple lobes, or sections, in two halves called hemispheres. The right and left hemispheres are divided by the medial longitudinal fissure. The *falx cerebrii* is a portion of the dura that resides in the medial longitudinal fissure. The two hemispheres are connected by the *corpus callosum*, a tract or bundle of axons extending horizontally, which facilitates communication between the two hemispheres (Figure 1.6).

The outer surface of the hemispheres is the cerebral cortex, an area made up primarily of the soma of neurons. The cerebral cortex

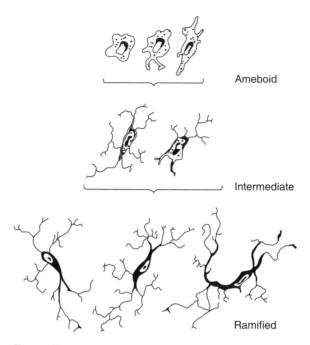

Fig. 1.4 The three main morphological aspects of microglial cells. Reprinted from Verney, C., Monier, A., Fallet-Bianco, C. and Gressens, P. (2010). Early microglial colonization of the human forebrain and possible involvement in periventricular white-matter injury of preterm infants. *Journal of Anatomy*, 217: 436–448. doi: 10.1111/j.1469-7580.2010.01245.x with permission from John Wiley & Sons, Inc.

is often referred to as gray matter because the nuclei within soma stain dark. The cortex contains many bulges called gyrus (plural gyri) and sulcus (plural sulci) as it folds to increase the surface area. The white matter lies beneath the cortex and contains mainly tracts, or groups of axons. Myelin covering many of the axons does not stain with older stains used during the early days of neuroanatomy exploration, hence the axon heavy areas are termed white matter.

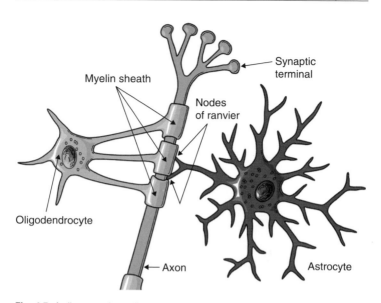

Fig. 1.5 A diagram of an oligodendrocyte. Courtesy of the Office of Communications and Public Liaison. (2002). *The life and death of a neuron* (NIH Publication No. 02-3440d). Bethesda, MD: National Institute of Neurological Disorders and Stroke at the National Institutes of Health.

Frontal lobe

The right and left frontal lobes are the anterior portion of the hemispheres (Figure 1.7). They are defined by the front edge of the hemisphere and the primary motor cortex, also called the primary motor strip or the precentral gyrus. The central sulcus lies immediately behind the precentral gyrus, separating the frontal lobe from the parietal lobe. The lateral sulcus, or sylvian fissure, separates the posterior portion of the frontal lobe from the temporal lobe.

The most anterior portion (approximately one-half) of the frontal lobe is termed the prefrontal lobe or prefrontal cortex. Neurons in this area initiate the planning of complex cognitive tasks, initiate decision making, inform personality expression, and moderate social behaviors. This area of the brain is thought to be responsible for goal-oriented behavior and high-level cognitive and abstract thinking.

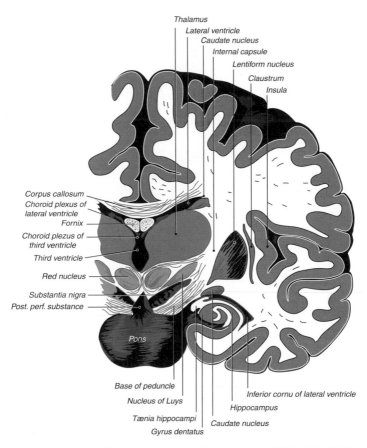

Fig. 1.6 A diagram of the diencephalon. Reprinted from Lewis, W. H. (Ed.). (1918). *Anatomy of the human body.* Philadelphia, PA: Lea & Febiger.

Other regions of the frontal lobe maintain long-term memory, motor function via the primary motor cortex, and speech production via Broca's area.

Parietal lobe

The parietal lobe is the portion of the brain behind the frontal lobe. It is separated from the frontal lobe by the central sulcus

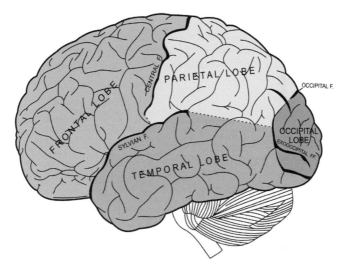

Fig. 1.7 A diagram of the lobes of the brain. Reprinted from Lewis, W. H. (Ed.). (1918). *Anatomy of the human body.* Philadelphia, PA: Lea & Febiger.

and extends to the parieto-occipital sulcus (immediately anterior to the occipital lobe) and down to the lateral sulcus, also called the Sylvian fissure, immediately above the temporal lobe. Adjacent to the primary motor strip of the frontal lobe, within the parietal lobe, lies the primary sensory cortex, also called the post-central gyrus or the somatosensory cortex. The primary sensory cortex is important to processing sensory input in the brain. Other portions of the parietal lobe are responsible for visuospatial processing, numerical knowledge and relations, and object recognition and manipulation.

Temporal lobe
The temporal lobe is the portion of the brain beneath the lateral sulcus/sylvian fissure extending to the anterior lower portion of the occipital lobe. The neurons in this region form the primary auditory cortex, which contains Wernicke's area and is responsible for hearing and speech processing, and the hippocampus, responsible for long-term memory formation. The inferior region of the temporal lobe also processes complex visual information such as facial recognition and object perception and recognition.

Occipital lobe

The occipital lobe is the most posterior portion of the cerebral cortex. This area of the brain houses neurons that process visual stimuli allowing vision, color perception, visual spatial processing, and motion perception.

Diencephalon structures

The diencephalon is the innermost aspect of the cerebral cortex. Structures within the diencephalons include the thalamus, hypothalamus, and the pituitary gland (Figure 1.9).

The thalamus surrounds the third ventricle and processes information between the cerebral cortex and the brain stem structures. Auditory, visual, gustatory, somatic, and somatosensory information are all processed in this area. Neurons within this region influence arousal and consciousness.

The hypothalamus lies inferior to the anterior portion of the thalamus. The hypothalamus serves to connect the cerebral cortex and the pituitary gland. Through hormonal stimulation of the pituitary gland the hypothalamus regulates body temperature and blood pressure. Hypothalamic input also plays a role in immune response, gastric reflexes, hunger, thirst, and circadian rhythms.

The pituitary gland dangles below the hypothalamus, connected via the pituitary stalk. It is structurally divided into two regions, the anterior and posterior, with different functions. The anterior pituitary gland releases hormones that modify blood pressure, gluceoneogenesis, immune response, metabolism, growth, lactation, ovulation, and reproductive functioning. The posterior pituitary gland releases hormones that modify fluid homeostasis and blood pressure and facilitate labor, birth, and lactation.

The basal ganglia is a region in the center of the brain, although formally it is part of the telencephalon (cerebral cortex/upper brain regions), not the diencephalons. The basal ganglia modify motor function by providing inhibitory input to the motor tracts, coordinating smooth movement.

Cerebellum

The cerebellum is a region of the brain that lies below the cerebral cortex and posterior to the brainstem structures. It is formally

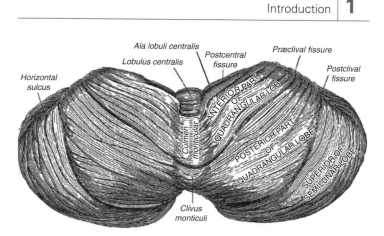

Fig. 1.8 A diagram of the cerebellum. Reprinted from Lewis, W. H. (Ed.). (1918). *Anatomy of the human body*. Philadelphia, PA: Lea & Febiger.

separated from the cerebral cortex by a layer of dura mater called the *tentorium cerebelli*. Neurons within the cerebellum receive input from the pons, brain, and spinal cord and send input to the pons and down the spinal cord to coordinate motor movement. Recent evidence has implicated the cerebellum in modifying language, attention, and mental imagery via connections with cerebral cortex (Figure 1.8).

Brainstem structures

The brainstem resides beneath the diencephalon, connecting the brain and the spinal cord. Sensory and motor tracts travel through the midbrains structures to the spinal cord, carrying impulses that stimulate motor movement or signal sensation. The midbrain is divided into three distinct areas: midbrain, pons, and medulla (Figure 1.9).

The midbrain is the uppermost portion of the brainstem, connecting the brain to the pons. The cerebral aquaduct – the small tube connecting the third and fourth ventricles – passes through the midbrain. Motor neurons and sensory neurons pass through this area. The midbrain houses many cranial nerves. It is involved in hearing, vision, arousal and consciousness, pain sensation, and

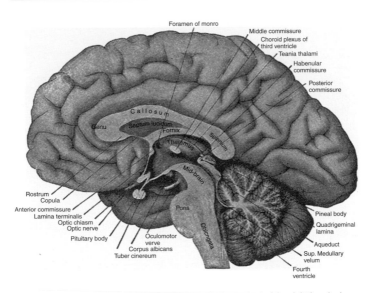

Fig. 1.9 A diagram of the brainstem structures in the context of the right hemisphere. Reprinted from Lewis, W. H. (Ed.). (1918). *Anatomy of the human body*. Philadelphia, PA: Lea & Febiger.

maintaining cardiovascular and respiratory homeostasis. Cranial nerves III and IV originate in the midbrain.

The pons lies between the midbrain (above) and medulla (below). Motor and sensory tracts pass through this region. Neurons within the pons send and receive input to/from the cerebellum. It has regions driving sleep, respiratory drive, swallowing, hearing, balance, bladder control, taste, eye movements, and facial expression and sensation. Cranial nerves V, VI, VII, and VIII originate in the pons.

The medulla is the region of the brainstem connecting pons and spinal cord. It provides stimulation to modify cardiovascular and respiratory homeostasis, and vomiting, coughing, sneezing, swallowing and balance. Cranial nerves IX, X, and XII originate in the medulla.

CEREBRAL BLOOD FLOW
Cerebral blood vessel structure
The blood vessels supplying blood to the brain have the same structure as they do in other regions of the body. The outermost layer of an artery is the *tunica externa* (or *adventitia*), made up of connective tissue. The *tunica media*, or middle layer, is made up of multiple layers of smooth muscle cells and elastic fibers. The smooth muscle cells of an artery respond to vasomotor modifiers to constrict or relax, altering the size of the internal lumen and modifying blood delivery to tissues. The most internal section of an artery, coming in direct contact with the blood and creating the internal lumen, is made up of a single layer of epithelial cells. Epithelial cells monitor the local environment and release nitric oxide and other vasomotor tone modifiers that modulate constriction and relaxation of the vessel, impacting blood flow delivery (see Figure 1.10).

BLOOD BRAIN BARRIER
The blood brain barrier serves to restrict passage of substances from the blood to the brain. This is vital to protect the CNS from infectious agents and toxins. The brain is very vulnerable to toxins, as neurons are not able to go through mitosis, so cell death results in permanent cell loss. It is also vulnerable to infectious agents, as immune cells are also provided restricted entry.

Major vessels
See Figure 1.11 for a schematic diagram of the cerebral vessels and the Circle of Willis.

ANTERIOR CIRCULATION
Internal carotid arteries
The right common carotid artery branches off from the brachiocephalic artery, while the left common carotid artery branches off from the arch of the aorta. The common carotid arteries travel up through the neck before branching off into the external and internal carotid arteries on either side of the neck. The right and left internal carotid arteries travel into the cranial cavity to the Circle of Willis. They bifurcate into the middle cerebral arteries and the anterior

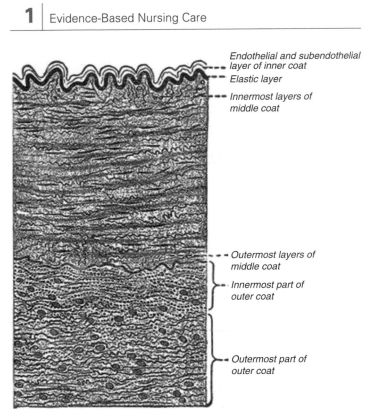

Endothelial and subendothelial layer of inner coat

Elastic layer

Innermost layers of middle coat

Outermost layers of middle coat

Innermost part of outer coat

Outermost part of outer coat

Fig. 1.10 A diagram of a cross-section of an artery. Reprinted from Lewis, W. H. (Ed.). (1918). *Anatomy of the human body.* Philadelphia, PA: Lea & Febiger.

cerebral arteries, thereby providing blood flow to the anterior and superior portions of the brain.

Middle cerebral arteries

The right and left middle cerebral arteries are formed by the internal carotid arteries. They continues through the center of the brain along the lateral sulcus where it branches and extends to a large portion of the cerebral cortex. The middle cerebral arteries supply blood to all but the most superior portion of the frontal and parietal lobes, the inferior portion of the temporal lobe, the internal capsule,

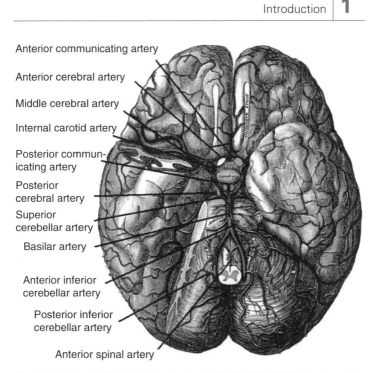

Anterior communicating artery

Anterior cerebral artery

Middle cerebral artery

Internal carotid artery

Posterior communicating artery

Posterior cerebral artery

Superior cerebellar artery

Basilar artery

Anterior inferior cerebellar artery

Posterior inferior cerebellar artery

Anterior spinal artery

Fig. 1.11 Circle of Willis. Reprinted from Lewis, W. H. (Ed.). (1918). *Anatomy of the human body*. Philadelphia, PA: Lea & Febiger.

and the basal ganglia. This area includes Broca's area, Wernicke's area, the motor cortex, the sensory cortex, the motor tracts and other structures within the brain.

Anterior cerebral arteries

The right and left anterior cerebral arteries branch off from the internal carotid arteries. They extend forward in the brain and provide blood to the medial portions of the frontal lobe, the medial/superior portions of the parietal lobe, the anterior portion of the corpus callosum, anterior portions of the basal ganglia and internal capsule, and the olfactory bulb and tract.

Anterior communicating artery

The anterior communicating artery connects the right and left anterior cerebral arteries. It does not supply blood directly to any area of the brain, but rather serves to ensure adequate blood flow to both hemispheres even in the presence of a lesion within the Circle of Willis.

POSTERIOR CIRCULATION

Vertebral arteries

There are a right and a left vertebral arteries. The vertebral arteries branch off from the subclavian arteries in the chest. They travel through the posterior neck and into the cranial vault. At the level of the midbrain, the two vertebral arteries merge to form the basilar artery.

Basilar artery

The basilar artery extends alongside the brainstem structures from the point where the vertebral arteries merge to the division into two posterior cerebral arteries. The posterior inferior cerebellar arteries (right and left), the anterior inferior cerebellar arteries, and the superior cerebellar arteries branch off from the basilar artery and supply blood to the cerebellum. There are several smaller arteries that branch off from the basilar artery, called the pontine arteries. The pontine arteries supply blood to the pons and other adjacent brainstem structures.

Posterior cerebral arteries

The posterior cerebral arteries (right and left) form at the top of the basilar artery. They have many smaller branching arteries that provide blood to the occipital lobe, the inferior portion of the temporal lobe, portions of the thalamus, the walls of the third ventricle, the caudate nucleus, and the cerebral peduncles.

Posterior communicating arteries

The posterior communicating arteries (left and right) serve to connect the posterior cerebral arteries and the trifurcation of the internal carotid arteries, the middle cerebral arteries, and the anterior cerebral arteries. The posterior communicating arteries connect anterior and posterior portions of the Circle of Willis, providing a mechanism for adequate blood delivery when lesions are present or all vessels of the Circle of Willis are not fully formed.

Circle of Willis

The Circle of Willis includes the anterior communicating artery, the anterior cerebral arteries, the internal carotid arteries, the posterior communicating arteries, and the posterior cerebral arteries. While clearly vital to cerebral blood flow, the middle cerebral arteries, basilar artery, and vertebral arteries are not considered part of the Circle of Willis (Figure 1.11).

The major vessels of the Circle of Willis branch off into smaller vessels and extend throughout all regions of the brain, providing adequate blood flow to the entire brain. When one vessel is not functioning properly due to injury or disease, collateral flow can provide some blood to the tissue at risk. This occurs because several branches overlap in the region of brain to which they provide blood. If a distal portion of the middle cerebral artery is damaged, some of the tissue it perfuses in normal circumstances will be perfused by nearby vessels from a different branch. If a central portion of the middle cerebral artery is damaged, a very large area of tissue will be deprived of blood flow and at risk for damage.

FACTORS INFLUENCING CEREBRAL BLOOD FLOW

Normal cerebral blood flow is 45–60 ml/100 g/min. The brain has considerable capacity to maintain adequate function with decreases in cerebral blood flow to about 20 ml/100 g/min, although electroencephalograph slowing and decrease in levels of consciousness are common at this level. When cerebral blood flow drops to less than 18 ml/100 g/min, anaerobic metabolism ensues and ionic/membrane homeostasis is impaired. At cerebral blood flow values of less than 10 ml/100 g/min, irreversible damage occurs as cellular membrane integrity is lost, calcium flows freely into the cell, and neuronal (and other) cell death occurs. Cerebral blood flow values less than 5 ml/100 g/min for more than 30 minutes, as may be seen in out-of-hospital cardiac arrest scenarios, leads to tissue infarction. Brain infarction may occur at higher cerebral blood flow values if maintained for longer periods of time. Cerebral blood flow of 10 ml/100 g/min can be tolerated for up to 3 hours and values of 18 ml/100 g/min may be tolerated for up to 4 hours. Normal cerebral metabolism – the amount of oxygen used by the brain – is between 1.3 and 1.8 μmol/g/min (Janigro et al., 1996; Ritter & Robertson, 1994).

Cerebral autoregulation is the concept according to which the brain receives adequate blood flow and nutrient delivery across a wide range of blood pressures. Within a range of mean arterial blood pressures between approximately 50 and 150 mm Hg, cerebral vasculature is able to dilate or constrict to regulate blood delivery to the tissues. When mean arterial blood pressure falls outside this range, blood flow is impaired. Mean arterial blood pressures below 50 mm Hg do not provide adequate force to perfuse the tissues. Mean arterial blood pressures greater than 150 mm Hg can lead to damage to the cerebral vasculature. Specifically, high blood pressure dilates the vessels and separates the tight endothelial junctions of the blood brain barrier, reducing its effectiveness.

Control of cerebral blood flow is impacted by several factors including metabolic demands of the brain, pressure within the skull, oxygen/carbon dioxide/H+/K/adenosine/prostaglandins/NO levels within the brain, and neural input. Each of these factors contributes varying influence on cerebral blood flow at different times. The following section discusses the influence of these factors individually.

Metabolic factors

The brain requires a near-constant supply of oxygen and glucose to maintain adequate energy for normal functioning. Individual cells within the central nervous system have a very limited capacity to store oxygen or glucose, and demands are high.

Glucose

The first step in both aerobic and anaerobic energy production is glycolysis, or the breakdown of glucose. Glucose is transported across the blood brain barrier by GLUT-1, a transporter molecule. It is taken up by astrocytes, via GLUT-1, and neurons, via glucose transporter GLUT-3. Intracellular glucose is broken down in the cytoplasm into 2 moles of pyruvate, 2 moles of nicotinamide adenine dinucleotide (NADH), and 4 moles of ATP. This reaction requires 2 moles of ATP, for a net yield of 2 moles of ATP. In the absence of oxygen, pyruvate is further broken down into lactate. In the presence of oxygen, pyruvate is converted into acetylcoenzyme A or oxaloacetate, which enter the mitochondria and are used in the Kreb's cycle and/or electron transport chain as part of oxidative metabolism. Without adequate glucose, glycolysis does not occur, NADH is not produced, and cellular-level energy failure quickly ensues.

Oxygen

Oxygen delivery to the brain is vital for maximal functioning. The brain has a very limited capacity for oxygen storage, and a constant supply is necessary. Oxygen is transported into the body, the blood, and ultimately to tissues by diffusion across the oxygen pressure gradient. The partial pressure of arterial oxygen is approximately 90 mm Hg and the partial pressure of cerebral oxygen is approximately 35 mm Hg. Oxygen is extracted from the air by alveoli of the lungs and transported directly to the blood where a large portion of it binds to hemoglobin. Oxygen remains bound to hemoglobin in the blood until it reaches capillaries and smaller vessels. In the small vessels and capillaries, the partial pressure of oxygen is lower in the tissue, and thus oxygen is released to the tissue.

Once in the tissue, oxygen is used to generate energy. Aerobic metabolism generates significantly more energy, or adenosine triphosphate (ATP), than anaerobic metabolism. Aerobic metabolism yields 36+ moles of ATP while anaerobic metabolism relies primarily on glycolysis and yields 2 moles of ATP. Adequate energy is important for neurons as it is the source of energy used by the cell to maintain homeostasis of the cell membrane (via pumps). While neurons are the CNS cell type most sensitive to oxygen deprivation, other CNS cell types are affected as well, with oligodendrocytes, astrocytes, and microglia being sensitive in that order.

Carbon dioxide

Carbon dioxide (and water) is generated as a by-product of aerobic metabolism. It has local effects that include vasodilation in an effort to increase oxygen delivery to the affected tissue and clear carbon dioxide. Ultimately, carbon dioxide modifies cerebral blood flow by altering local pH. In the tissue, carbon dioxide reacts with water to generate bicarbonate and hydrogen ($H+$). High amounts of carbon dioxide result in an acidotic environment, which dilates blood vessels and increases cerebral blood flow to local tissues.

Nitric oxide

Nitric oxide is a strong vasodilator produced within the central nervous system and at the neurovascular junction. Nitric oxide is produced by its cleavage from L-arginine by nitric oxide synthase (NOS). Neurons and glia produce nNOS, endothelial cells produce eNOS, and other cells produce inducible NOS (iNOS). Endothelial cells and neurons and glia near the vasculature produce NOS in response to low blood flow or increased metabolic needs. The locally produced NOS quickly generates nitric oxide, which dilates the local cerebral blood vessels. While nitric oxide has beneficial effects through vasodilation, it also interacts with free radicals, and overproduction may lead to further damage.

Adenosine

Adenosine is released during the breakdown/use of ATP. Adenosine is required for cyclic-adenosine monophosphate (cAMP) production, which increases cerebral blood flow. In periods of hypoxia, adenosine is produced by local astrocytes. Adenosine actives nitric oxide release, which causes vasodilation (Zauner et al., 2002).

Cerebral acid-base balance

Acidotic blood promotes oxygen extraction from the blood by tissues, while alkalotic blood inhibits oxygen extraction from the blood. In anaerobic conditions, lactate accumulates in local tissues and generates a hydrogen-rich, acidic extracellular environment. During normal cellular functioning, lactate accumulation and an acidotic intracellular environment do not appear to be detrimental. However, in periods of cellular-level stress, such as hypoxia or ischemia, the accumulation of lactate and an acidotic environment leads to intracellular buffering systems becoming exhausted, which in turn leads to cellular-level damage from neuronal denatured proteins, astrocytic membrane transport system failure, free radical formation, and inhibition of glycolysis. In hypoxic and ischemic states, carbon dioxide retention and ATP breakdown occurs, further contributing to the acidotic state. Sodium/hydrogen exchange transporters are activated in acidotic intracellular states that control some of the damage; however, this activation has also been shown to cause CNS tissue swelling and edema.

Temperature
Local brain temperature has a direct influence on metabolic needs of the brain. Under conditions of hyperthermia, metabolic needs increase as individual cells attempt to maintain ionic balance. Under conditions of hypothermia, metabolic needs are decreased and less oxygen is released from the blood to the tissue.

Pressure
On the most basic level, cerebral blood flow is modified by pressures within the arterial system and the intracranial space. Maintaining adequate cerebral blood flow and perfusion of the cerebral tissue are paramount to brain functioning. Mean arterial blood pressure must be strong enough to push blood into the cranial vault and to the tissue. Normal mean arterial blood pressure ranges from 70 to 100 mm Hg. Intracranial pressure, or the pressure within the cranial vault, provides a form of resistance to the blood pressure. Normal intracranial pressure is 10–15 mm Hg. Cerebral perfusion pressure is the pressure required to deliver blood to the tissues and is defined clinically as mean arterial pressure minus intracranial pressure. Normal cerebral perfusion pressure is 70–100 mm Hg. As intracranial volume increases, either by an increase mass (e.g., tumor, edema) or fluid (e.g., extracerebral hemorrhage or cerebrospinal fluid), the intracranial pressure rises. With an increase in intracranial pressure, blood pressure needs to increase to maintain adequate perfusion pressure. In conditions where mean arterial blood pressure is very low, as in cardiac arrest situations, cerebral perfusion pressure becomes low and tissue may suffer the effects of inadequate cerebral blood flow, mainly hypoxia and ischemia.

Neural input
The cerebral vessels are innervated with sympathetic nerve fibers and trigeminal nerve fibers. Inputs from these neurons are minimal under normal conditions; however, it may have a more significant influence in conditions of abnormal blood pressure and/or brain functioning.

REFERENCES

Janigro, D., Wender, R., Ransom, G., Tinklepaugh, D. L., & Winn, H. R. (1996). Adenosine-induced release of nitric oxide from cortical astrocytes. *Neuroreport*, *7*(10), 1640–1644.

Ritter, A. M., & Robertson C. S. (1994). Cerebral metabolism. *Neurosurgery Clinics of North America*, *5*(4), 633–645.

Zauner, A., Daugherty, W. P., Bullock, M. R., & Warner, D. S. (2002). Brain oxygenation and energy metabolism: Part I – biological function and pathophysiology. *Neurosurgery*, *51*(2), 289–301; discussion 302.

Transient Ischemic Attacks

2

Lori M. Massaro

Evidence-Based Nursing Care for Stroke and Neurovascular Conditions,
First Edition. Edited by Sheila A. Alexander.
© 2013 John Wiley & Sons, Inc. Published 2013 by John Wiley & Sons, Inc.

DEFINITION

Recently released professional statements and guidelines have contributed to a refined definition and recommendations for patients who present with transient ischemic attacks (TIA). The most recent definition incorporates brain imaging, specifically the presence or absence of infarction as a component of the data necessary for final diagnosis. Transient ischemic attack is defined as a brief episode of neurological dysfunction caused by focal brain, spinal cord, or retinal ischemia with no evidence of infarction on brain imaging. The clinical characterization of TIA, spinal cord ischemia and retinal ischemia, often manifested as amaurosis fugax (transient loss of vision in one eye), were published in the AHA/ASA scientific statement on the definition and evaluation of TIA (Easton et al., 2009). Historically, TIA was defined by the duration of the neurologic symptoms and broadly included patients who experience complete resolution of neurologic symptoms within 24 hours. However, many of us who specialize in stroke have encountered patients with complete resolution of clinical stroke symptoms, but find MRI and/or CT findings consistent with an acute cerebral infarction or stroke. This paradigm shift from time- to tissue-based diagnosis encourages practitioners to utilize diagnostic neuroimaging to determine if infarction has occurred, to further support the final diagnosis of TIA. The recognition and diagnosis of TIA signals a need to further evaluate for known preventable causes of ischemic stroke and an opportunity to intervene in order to prevent a potentially disabling stroke.

EPIDEMIOLOGY

Accurate information on the incidence and prevalence of TIA is difficult to calculate because of the varying clinical presentations and criteria to collect this data. It is suspected that the currently available statistics underestimate the actual impact and prevalence of TIA. This is suspected because of lack of symptom recognition and under-reporting by patients who do not seek immediate medical care, coupled with the lack of accurate diagnostic criteria that has been used by healthcare providers.

The reported incidence of TIA increases with age and varies by race/ethnicity. According to the most recent data published by the AHA/ASA, the incidence is estimated to be in the range of

200,000–500,000 per year (Easton et al., 2009). In patients who present with stroke, the percentage of patients who report prior TIA ranges from 7% to 40% (Bogousslavsky, Van Melle, & Regli, 1988). In the Northern Manhattan Stroke Study, the prevalence of TIA's was found to be 8.7%, with the majority of TIAs having occurred within the preceding 30 days of the patient's first ischemic stroke. Forty-one percent of the patients in this study reported a TIA that lasted longer than 1 hour in duration (Sacco, 2004).

PATHOPHYSIOLOGY

The primary mechanism of neuronal or retinal ischemia is arterial occlusion resulting in lack of oxygen delivery to the cells responsible for the specific area of neurologic function. Ischemia can be partial or complete. Partial ischemia may cause hypoxia that results in too little oxygen reaching the cells and/or tissue. Complete ischemia results in anoxia, where no oxygen reaches the target cells and tissue. Without restoration of arterial blood supply to the area, cerebral infarction or a stroke will eventually result. The brain functions at a high metabolic rate that is supported by high volume of constant blood supply. Research over the years has provided a variety of definitions and time frames at which brain cells can remain viable while enduring low flow states. Because of the high metabolic demands for cerebral functioning, 15% of the total cardiac output is supplied to the brain for cerebral blood flow, equating to 50–54 ml of blood per 100 g of brain tissue per minute. Ischemia results if the cerebral blood flow falls below 18–20 ml/mg brain/min, and neuronal tissue death occurs if blood flow is sustained at or below 8–10 mg/100 g brain/minute.

PHYSIOLOGIC CAUSES

The physiologic causes of TIA and stroke are largely the same. A more in-depth review of stroke etiology will be covered in the next chapter on ischemic stroke. For the purposes of the more detailed explanation of TIA, the etiology is divided into three categories: large artery atherosclerosis, embolic, and small vessel disease.

Large artery atherosclerosis of the anterior and posterior cerebral vessels results from progressive accumulation of plaque within the vessel wall, producing a reduction in the luminal diameter. This process is similar to what is now believed to be the pathophysiology and etiology of coronary artery disease. Common vessels at risk of atherosclerosis are located in both intracranial and extracranial arterial segments. These include the vertebral arteries (origins to intracranial segments), basilar artery, internal carotid artery (bifurcation to intracranial segments), and middle cerebral artery.

Embolic TIA can occur if an embolus, originating elsewhere in the body, dislodges and then enters the cerebral circulation via the large arteries of the anterior and posterior circulation. The clot becomes lodged when it exceeds the vessel diameter, causing vessel occlusion and eventual ischemia in the area of the brain supplied by the occluded artery. A common source of cerebral embolism is a cardiac etiology. Cardioembolism is responsible for approximately 20% of all ischemic strokes. Arial fibrillation, valvular heart disease, and left ventricular mural thrombus in the setting of reduced ejection fraction are the most common cardiac abnormalities associated with embolus formation.

Small vessel disease or penetrating artery disease occurs in the smaller arteries of the brain because of caliber modifications and arteriolar wall modifications that produce intimal thickening. The vessel wall becomes sclerotic and sometimes hyalinotic (a translucent albuminoid substance, one of the products of amyloid degeneration). Microangiopathy is associated in variable proportions with sclerosis, hyalinosis, and lipid deposits. It is characterized by disorganization of the vessel wall and disappearance of the smooth muscles (Welch et al., 1997). The diagnosis of small vessel strokes is largely determined by the presence of periventricular white matter changes seen on CT or flair sequence of MRI and accompanying clinical diagnoses of hypertension, hyperlipidemia, diabetes, and smoking. Imaging of the small penetrating vessels is difficult and has not been achieved by conventional angiography or CT angiography. Radiographically, the most common locations of small vessel stroke are in the basal ganglia, coronal radiate, internal capsule, thalamus, and pons.

An additional physiologic cause of TIA or transient neurologic dysfunction is related to a hypoperfusion syndrome that may occur with sudden onset of cardiac dysrhythmia, vasovagal reaction, or glucose deprivation states that may result from hypoglycemia. On correction of the initial inciting nidus (hypotension, arrhythmia, hypoglycemia), the blood flow is restored and transient neurologic symptoms resolve. Syncope is defined as a sudden impairment of intracranial blood flow resulting from hypotension, cardiac arrhythmia, or cardiac outflow obstruction. Syncope is completely and rapidly reversible.

PREVENTION

Prevention of TIA is largely dependent on risk factor identification and medical or surgical management to reduce discovered risks. Atrial fibrillation, carotid disease, hypertension, and hyperlipidemia are frequent risk factors. A more in-depth discussion of prevention strategies base on etiology will be included in the subsequent chapter on stroke (see Chapter 3).

DIAGNOSIS

Any patient who develops transient neurologic symptoms should be advised to seek immediate medical attention. An evaluation by a trained health care professional to determine the severity and duration of symptoms, medical history, and to perform a thorough neurologic exam is advised. A diagnostic evaluation can be expedited by the use of TIA clinics where available (Bogousslavsky, Van Melle, & Regli, 1988). The use of TIA clinics has increased in the past several years, and these are usually staffed by neurologists and advanced practice nurses. Collaboration with diagnostic services is necessary to accomplish an expedited assessment of treatable risk factors for stroke. An alternative for an expedited assessment is for the patient to be admitted to the hospital for 23-hour observation, with an organized pathway to direct care and to obtain critical diagnostic testing within the specified time period.

Additionally, some physician groups and emergency departments are now using the ABCD2 scoring system to risk-stratify patients and determine the need for urgent diagnostic evaluation. The ABCD2 score was developed and tested, with results published in the *Lancet* in 2007 (see Table 2.1) (Johnston et al., 2007). This scoring system is used to collect critical data about the neurologic symptoms and accompanying risks. Data collected to calculate the ABCD2 score includes age, blood pressure at the time of assessment, clinical features of the TIA/neurologic symptoms and duration, and presence of diabetes. The scores are summed and

Table 2.1 ABCD2 score

Age ≥ 60	If yes = 1 point
Blood Pressure ≥ 140/90 mmHg on first evaluation	If yes = 1 point
Clinical symptoms include focal weakness at time of T IA	If yes = 2 points
Clinical symptoms include speech impairment without weakness	If yes = 1 point
Duration of symptoms ≥ 60 minutes	If yes = 2 points
10 − 59 minutes	If yes = 1 point
	Total score _____

Johnson S. C., Rothwell, P. M., Nguyer-Huynh, M. N., Giles, M. F., Elkins, J. S., Bernstein, A. L., & Sidney, S. (2007). Validation and refinement of scores to predict very early stroke risk after transient ischaemic attack. *Lancet, 369*, 283–292.

two-day stroke risk can be determined based on the data from this trial. (See Table 2.2 for risk/recommendations.)

DIAGNOSTIC TESTING RECOMMENDED

Diagnostic testing may be tailored to first assess the presumed or most likely TIA/stroke etiology. The goal of obtaining early brain imaging is obtained to determine if an infarction has occurred, and to identify if vessel stenosis or occlusion are present, which may increase the risk of impending ischemic stroke. Both computed tomography (CT) and magnetic resonance imaging (MRI) are used, but there is a higher degree of sensitivity for early ischemic changes when using MRI.

Non-contrasted CT of the brain is more readily available and can be accomplished within relatively short periods of time on an

Table 2.2 ABCD2 Risk stratification – guidelines

Total score – then reference 2-day stroke risk	
0%	for scores 0–1
1.3%	for scores 2–3
4.1%	for scores 4–5
8.1%	for scores 6–7

Johnson S. C., Rothwell, P. M., Nguyer-Huynh, M. N., Giles, M. F., Elkins, J. S., Bernstein, A. L., & Sidney, S. (2007). Validation and refinement of scores to predict very early transient ischaemic attack. *Lancet, 369*,283–292.

urgent basis. It is the most widely available test and is recommended in patients with contraindication for MRI to determine if ischemic changes are present – ischemic changes can be reported as loss of gray/white matter differentiation. This early change occurs because there is an increase in the water concentration within the ischemic tissues. With improved technology and multi-detector CT scanners, the detection of early ischemic changes on CT has improved, but there is still a chance that ischemic changes may lag and not be present within first 24 hours of symptoms.

MRI of the brain with Diffusion Weighted Imaging (DWI) sequencing is now commonly used to determine if acute ischemia is present. The DWI sequence may be positive within minutes of an ischemic event occurring. This change occurs because of the ischemic cellular cascade. This change is called restricted diffusion because extracellular water moves into the intracellular environment during ischemia. As a result, there is swelling of the cells and narrowing of the extracellular spaces. The isotropic DWI map makes abnormal areas of ischemia readily visible. Barber et al. demonstrated 100% sensitivity to ischemia with DWI versus 75% with CT within 6 hours (Barber et al., 1999).

Vessel assessment to stratify risk of stroke

Carotid Ultrasound (CUS) – limited to extracranial carotid assessment by velocity of flow through vessel. Unable to determine intracranial vessel status and velocity of flow in extracranial vertebrals.

Transcranial Doppler (TCD) – provided information regarding intracranial stenosis.

Magnetic Resonance Angiography (MRA) of head and neck – to determine vessel patency.

Computed Tomographic Angiography (CTA) of head and neck – to evaluate for stenosis, occlusion, and flow limitations.

Embolic etiologies

12-lead electrocardiogram (ECG) – to determine rhythm.

Extended monitoring – 24-, 48-, 30-day event monitors – to detect paroxysmal atrial fibrillation.

Transthoracic echocardiogram (TTE) – to evaluate left ventricle (LV) size and function, ejection fraction (EF), and rule out valvular anomalies.
Transesophageal echocardiogram (TEE) – to evaluate LV size and function, EF rule out valvular anomalies with greater detail.

Laboratory assessment
Fasting lipid profile
HgA1C
Treatment – aimed at prevention of ischemic stroke and is dependent on initial findings.
If embolic etiology is suspected – may need to initiate anticoagulant therapy acutely.
If thrombotic etiology is suspected – initiate antiplatelet therapy and risk factor modification to address hyperlipidemia, hypertension, diabetes, smoking cessation, ideal body mass, activity, and diet.

REFERENCES

Barber, P. A., Darby, D. G., Desmond, P. M., et al. (1999). Identification of major ischemic change. Diffusion-weighted imaging versus computed tomography. *Stroke, 30*(10), 2059–2065.
Bogousslavsky, J., Van Melle, G., & Regli, F. (1988). The Lausanne Stroke Registry: Analysis of 1,000 consecutive patients with first stroke. *Stroke, 19*(9), 1083–1092.
Easton, J. D., Saver, J. L., Albers, G. W., et al. (2009). Definition and evaluation of transient ischemic attack: A scientific statement for healthcare professionals from the American Heart Association/American Stroke Association Stroke Council; Council on Cardiovascular Surgery and Anesthesia; Council on Cardiovascular Radiology and Intervention; Council on Cardiovascular Nursing; and the Interdisciplinary Council on Peripheral Vascular Disease. The American Academy of Neurology affirms the value of this statement as an educational tool for neurologists. *Stroke, 40*(6), 2276–2293.
Johnston, S. C., Rothwell, P. M., Nguyen-Huynh, M. N., et al. (2007). Validation and refinement of scores to predict very early

stroke risk after transient ischaemic attack. *Lancet*, *369*(9558), 283–292.

Sacco, R. L. (2004). Risk factors for TIA and TIA as a risk factor for stroke. *Neurology*, *62*(8 Suppl 6), S7–S11.

Welch, K. M. A., Caplan, L. R., Reis, D. J., Siesjo, B. K., & Weir, B. (eds). (1997). *Primer on cerebrovascular diseases*. New York: Academic Press.

Ischemic Stroke

3

Lori M. Massaro

Evidence-Based Nursing Care for Stroke and Neurovascular Conditions,
First Edition. Edited by Sheila A. Alexander.
© 2013 John Wiley & Sons, Inc. Published 2013 by John Wiley & Sons, Inc.

DEFINITION

The improved recognition of symptoms, acute treatment options, and emphasis on prevention of recurrent stroke has evolved at a rapid pace over the past 15 years. The definition of TIA has been revised and now excludes patient with acute neuroimaging findings revealing ischemia even if the clinical symptoms have resolved. This change has shifted some formerly classified TIA patients into the category of ischemic stroke. By definition, an ischemic stroke is the result of neuronal death due to lack of oxygen, which leads to focal brain injury. Radiographically, this is accompanied by tissue changes consistent with an infarction found on neuroimaging of the central nervous system tissue. Strokes may be accompanied by clinical symptoms or may occur in the absence of clinical findings and be considered clinically silent.

PREVALENCE/INCIDENCE

Stroke affects approximately 795,000 Americans each year, and there are estimated to be 6.4 million stroke survivors in the United States (Writing Group M et al., 2010). Progress had been made in reducing mortality associated with stroke and recently it has fallen one ranking to claim the fourth leading cause of death in the United States. Stroke is the leading cause of disability, with 20% of survivors requiring institutional care after 3 months and 15–30% having permanent disability (Writing Group M et al., 2010). Stroke is a life-changing event that affects not only the survivor of the stroke, but also has a great impact on family members and caregivers.

ACUTE MEDICAL EVENTS THAT RESULT IN CEREBRAL ISCHEMIA

Cardiac arrest

Sudden cardiac arrest results in cessation of blood flow to the entire body including the brain. This results in global tissue hypoxia and oftentimes leads to cerebral ischemia. The goal of emergency care is directed at general return of spontaneous circulation (ROSC). Less than 8% of individuals who suffer cardiac arrest outside of the hospital survive the event, and many of those are individuals who have no known heart disease or risk factors (American Heart Association, 2010). Unless CPR and/or defibrillation are provided by witnessed observers within minutes of a collapse, it is unlikely that the resuscitation efforts will succeed. In addition to stroke, a variety of neurologic complications can result from global hypoxemia associated with cardiac arrest. Different areas of the brain seem more susceptible to hypoxia, with neurons in the hippocampus, cerebellum, striatum, and cerebral cortex appearing most vulnerable (Welch et al., 1997). Clinically, following cardiac arrest, patients are often described as being unconscious or comatose. In patients who demonstrate rapid neurologic improvement, the prognosis for recovery is better than for those who do not show improvement. The most common findings on computed tomography (CT) after cardiac arrest include diffuse swelling and inversion of gray/white matter densities. Magnetic resonance imaging (MRI) findings include diffuse high-intensity changes on diffusion weighted imaging (DWI) sequence that are suggestive of tissue ischemia (Young, 2009).

Treatment of recognized and/or witnessed cardiac arrest is first aimed at restoring circulation. The approval and availability of automated external defibrillators (AEDs) have impacted previously reported poor initial survival rates. After cardiac arrest, when a spontaneous cardiac rhythm is established, induced hypothermia is often initiated as a neuroprotective treatment. Cooling results in the reduction of cerebral metabolic demands and is thought to reduce the risk of ischemic injury to tissue following a period of insufficient blood flow (Yenari et al., 2008).

Drowning
Drowning occurs when water enters the lungs and causes asphyxia. During this time, the patient is unable to exchange and absorb oxygen, and the result, if left uncorrected, is cerebral hypoxia (Lunetta & Modell, 2005). In the absence of oxygen delivery to sustain metabolism, cellular ischemia followed by cell death results. In the case of drowning, the ischemia pattern is diffuse widespread and usually results in brain death.

Strangulation
Cerebral ischemia may occur in the setting of strangulation due to mechanical compression of the neck. This can result in brain ischemia by several mechanisms. First, compression of the carotid arteries prevents arterial blood flow to the brain; second, compression of the larynx or trachea prevents air entry into the lungs. A third

physiologic effect of strangulation involves the stimulation of the carotid sinus that can result in both bradycardia and hypotension. The combined results of these three processes are cerebral ischemia and neuronal death (Jones, 2006).

Choking

Choking is a result of a mechanical obstruction preventing movement of air from the mouth into the lungs. This leads to an inability to breathe, the cessation of oxygen exchange, and eventual asphyxia if the obstruction is not relieved. Left untreated, cerebral ischemia will result. The physical obstruction by a foreign body is the most commonly seen and recognized cause of choking. This should be treated if a bystander or witness is trained and able to perform the Heimlich maneuver in combination with back slaps (American Medical Association, 2009). Other causes of choking include compression of the larynx or trachea that was previously described in the strangulation section. Respiratory diseases that involve bronchospasm or obstruction of the airway can also result in choking. Cerebral ischemia is a late result if the obstruction is not relieved or if an artificial airway is not inserted to allow passage of air and exchange of oxygen/carbon dioxide.

Closed head injury

Mechanical trauma involving the head may also result in cerebral ischemia. The term "cerebral contusion" is often used to describe the injury that results when the head is struck by an object or otherwise forcefully receives an external blow. This type of closed head injury results in bruising of the brain tissue. The most common locations for contusions to be seen on imaging are in the frontal and temporal lobes. The most widely accepted explanation for these locations and the mechanism is that there is incongruent movement of the brain tissue on the bony structures of the cranium. The cranium is made up of bone that is not always characterized by a smooth inner surface. In coup and contra-coup types of injury patterns, the brain meets hard resistance with these inner bony areas of the cranium, and the brain tissue may bleed or swell in response.

Another mechanism of cerebral ischemia in the setting of trauma and closed head injury is diffuse axonal injury. This type of injury is seen in acceleration/deceleration situations and is not necessarily the result of a direct impact to the skull. When head trauma results in diffuse axonal injury, the axons are stretched and damaged as parts of the brain with different densities slide or shear over each other.

Following closed head injury that results from a contusion or diffuse axonal injury, edema often occurs. If the edema and tissue expansion exceed the capacity of the limited cranium size, increased intracranial pressure results. The consequences of untreated increased intracranial pressure (ICP) are reduction in arterial blood flow, compression of normal or uninjured tissue, and limited flow of cerebrospinal fluid (CSF) through the normal circulating pathways. Local or global cerebral ischemia results if ICP is not treated or relieved.

Carbon monoxide poisoning

Carbon monoxide is a colorless and odorless gas, toxic to humans. It is a by-product of faulty furnaces, older motor vehicles, and propane- or gasoline-powered appliances and tools. Physiologically, the mechanism of injury in humans is related to the inability of oxygen to bind to the hemoglobin molecule because the carbon monoxide molecule binds in its place. This results in reduced oxygen-carrying capacity of the blood, and, if sustained, generalized hypoxia results. As described earlier, prolonged systemic hypoxia affects cerebral function and may result in cerebral ischemia (Prockop & Chichkova, 2007). Treatment of carbon monoxide exposure or poisoning is to immediately remove the source and supply supplemental 100% oxygen.

CHRONIC CAUSES OF ISCHEMIC STROKE

Cerebral ischemia or stroke is often classified by the underlying pathophysiologic cause using the TOAST criteria (see Table 3.1).

Table 3.1 TOAST Criteria

Large artery atherosclerosis (LAA)
Cardioembolism (CE)
Small artery occlusion (SAO)
Acute stroke of other determined etiology (ASODE)
Stroke of undetermined etiology (SUE)

Major stroke trials and clinical practice guidelines refer to this criteria to classify the mechanism or cause of an ischemic stroke after completion and review of diagnostic testing following the initial stroke presentation. The TOAST criteria were initially tested and validated by Adams et al. (1993). Since that time the system has been widely adopted and used in the literature. Estimates of the breakdown of ischemic stroke by TOAST subtype was described by Albers et al. (2004). This report suggests that 20% if ischemic strokes are caused by large artery atherosclerosis (LAA), 20% are caused by cardioembolism (CE), 25% are caused by small artery occlusion (SAO), and 30% are strokes of undetermined etiology (SUE). The remaining 5% of strokes can be categorized in the acute stroke of other determined etiology (ASODE) category. These percentages may vary slightly by geographic differences within the United States.

Pathophysiology by subclassification of ischemic stroke
Thrombotic

An ischemic stroke is classified as thrombotic when there is evidence of artery stenosis or occlusion on vessel imaging, or if brain imaging suggests small vessel ischemic changes. The major large arteries that supply the cerebral circulation (carotid artery, middle cerebral artery, anterior cerebral artery, posterior cerebral artery, vertebral artery, or basilar artery) can develop luminal changes caused by plaque accumulation in both the intracranial and extracranial segments. Additionally, small arterial occlusions of the intracranial vessels that supply the deep structures of the brain and pons are considered thrombotic. Advances in neuroimaging have led to improved detection of vessel stenosis and/or occlusion. Testing by computed tomography angiography (CTA), magnetic resonance angiography (MRA), or carotid ultrasound (CUS) is recommended in the diagnostic evaluation after a patient presents with clinical symptoms consistent with stroke.

Large artery atherosclerosis of the anterior and posterior cerebral vessels results from progressive accumulation of plaque within the vessel wall producing reduction in the luminal diameter. This process is similar to what is well documented and recognized as the pathophysiology and etiology of coronary artery disease and peripheral vascular disease. The process found in arteries with occlusion or stenosis is complex and includes combined chronic and acute phases. The inciting process that results in vessel occlusion or embolus formation and subsequent clinical symptoms usually involves a thrombus overlying a pre-existing atherosclerotic plaque (Alsheikh-Ali et al., 2010). Many research efforts have focused on describing the mechanism, and it is generally accepted that there are both systemic and local factors that contribute to the process. Increased platelet reactivity and coagulation, pro-thrombotic substances, tissue factor, and glycoprotein IV activation all contribute to the process of thrombus formation in vulnerable plaques (Reininger et al., 2010).

When there is an acute occlusion of a cerebral artery, the tissue that is normally dependent on the constant blood supply is at risk for ischemia. Advances in both the acute and long-term management of large artery disease are discussed in the treatment portion of this chapter.

Small vessel disease or penetrating artery disease occurs in the smaller arteries of the brain resulting in caliber modifications and arteriolar wall modifications that produce intimal thickening. The vessel wall undergoes changes and becomes sclerotic and sometimes hyalinotic (a translucent albuminoid substance, one of the products of amyloid degeneration). Microangiopathy or disease of the small arteries of the brain is associated in with sclerosis, hyalinosis, and lipid deposits. These changes result in disorganization of the vessel wall and disappearance or reduction in the smooth muscles of the smaller vessel walls (Welch et al., 1997). The imaging diagnosis of small vessel strokes is often challenging and can be determined by the presence of periventricular white matter changes seen on CT or flair sequence of MRI and accompanying clinical risk factors of hypertension, hyperlipidemia, diabetes, and smoking (Welch et al., 1997). Imaging of the small penetrating vessels is difficult and has not been achieved by conventional digital subtraction angiography or CT angiography. Radiographically, the most common locations of small vessel stroke are in the basal ganglia, coronal radiata, internal capsule, thalamus, and pons (Welch et al., 1997).

Clinically, the presentation of patients with small artery occlusion differs from those with large artery occlusion. Small artery occlusions in the anterior circulation typically result in subcortical strokes that are manifested in pure motor or sensory symptoms, clumsy hand, dysarthria, or ataxia. It is rare to observe a small vessel stroke and see accompanying aphasia, visual field deficits, or neglect syndromes. In contrast, in the setting of a large artery stroke, there can be a variety of clinical presentations depending on the location, cerebral dominance, presence of collateral flow, patency of vessels of the Circle of Willis, and blood pressure as it relates to cerebral perfusion pressure.

Embolic

An embolic stroke occurs when a blood clot originating elsewhere in the body dislodges and then enters the cerebral circulation via the large arteries of the anterior and posterior circulation. The clot becomes lodged when it exceeds the vessel diameter, causing vessel occlusion and eventual ischemia in the area of the brain supplied by the occluded artery. Recognized sources of cerebral embolism include both artery-to-artery embolism and cardiac embolism.

An artery-to-artery embolism can develop in the setting of large artery atherosclerotic plaque or arterial dissection. With insufficient forward flow and intimal luminal abnormalities present, a thrombus is more likely to form. When a portion of the plaque, clot, or thrombus becomes dislodged, it then can serve as an embolic source of stroke as it travels into the cerebral circulation.

Arterial dissection is a less common cause of stroke and may be associated with neck trauma. In the setting of trauma, there is injury to the inner layer of the blood vessel wall and hematoma formation within this space that can be severe enough to result in vessel occlusion or severe stenosis. An additional cause of vessel dissection involves iatrogenic catheter injury that may occur during cerebral angiography. In either case, because of partial or complete occlusion, thrombus formation and embolization poses an increased risk in the setting of either carotid or vertebral artery dissection.

Cardioembolism is responsible for approximately 20% of all ischemic strokes. Arial fibrillation, valvular heart disease, left ventricular mural thrombus in the setting of reduced ejection fraction, atrial myxoma, mechanical prosthetic valves, and paradoxical emboli are the most common cardiac abnormalities that are associated with embolus formation that can lead to cerebral embolism and ischemic stroke (Furie et al., 2011). When an embolus originates in the heart, it can travel through the cardiac cycle and then be ejected from the left ventricle. The embolus then enters the cerebral circulation via the carotid arteries that originate in the aortic arch or into the vertebral arteries via the subclavian arteries. Clinical manifestations of arterial occlusion from a cardiac embolus vary depending on the location of occlusion and availability of collateral flow.

Hypercoagulability/Thrombophilia

Thrombophilia refers to tendency to form clots. In the setting of ischemic stroke, a thromboembolism may result if there are hematologic clotting abnormalities that predispose an individual to premature clotting. There are documented inherited and acquired thrombophilias that are associated with venous thrombosis, arterial thrombosis, and ischemic stroke. Primary thrombophilic states are thought to be responsible for 1–4% of all ischemic strokes (Ng, Loh, & Sharma, 2011). Examples of acquired thrombophilia states include the presence of antiphospholipid antibodies (aPL). This broader category includes both anticardiolipin antibody and lupus anticoagulant factor elevations that can be detected via serum screening. Young women with ischemic stroke have been found to have a higher prevalence of aPL. It is also known that the prevalence of aPL increases with age in both sexes.

Inherited or genetic causes of thrombophilia include abnormal Factor V Leiden mutation, the presence of prothrombin G20210A gene mutation, and protein C and S deficiencies (Goldstein et al., 2011). It is estimated that approximately 50% of the inherited causes of thrombophilia are due to Factor V Leiden mutation. Prothrombin gene mutations that are found in patients with cryptogenic stroke and patent Foramen Ovale (PFO) may be associated with venous thromboembolism. This can result in ischemic stroke when a thrombus from the venous circulation paradoxically shunts to the left side of the heart, becoming an arterial thrombus.

STROKE PREVENTION
Embolic stroke prevention

The most common source of an embolic stroke is atrial fibrillation. Chronic and paroxysmal atrial fibrillation represent common causes of initial and recurrent stroke. In the United States, fewer than 75,000 strokes per year are caused by atrial fibrillation, and it is estimated that over 2 million Americans are affected by atrial fibrillation (Furie et al., 2011). In the absence of cardiac valvular disease, there is a 4–5-fold increase in the risk of ischemic stroke in the setting of atrial fibrillation (Kannel & Benjamin, 2008). The recognition and diagnosis of chronic and paroxysmal atrial fibrillation is an important factor in primary stroke prevention, and electrocardiogram (ECG) screening of patients age 65 or older in the primary care setting is recommended (Goldstein et al., 2011). The use of the CHADS2 score has helped practitioners determine the risk/benefit ratio when considering anticoagulation for stroke prevention in this high risk group (Gage et al., 2001). Associated medical conditions that contribute to higher CHADS2 scores include congestive heart failure, hypertension, age 75 and older, diabetes, and stroke/TIA. Patients with a calculated CHADS2 score of 2 or greater are considered at moderate risk for stroke. Anticoagulation to prevent thrombus formation in the left atrial appendage is the recommended treatment for patients with risk of stroke related to atrial fibrillation.

The detection and accurate diagnosis of atrial fibrillation is often challenging. During the acute phase of stroke, continuous cardiac monitoring is indicated to assess rhythm and rule out arrhythmias. Extended cardiac monitoring following discharge is often ordered in situations where the stroke is thought to be of embolic origin, but no rhythm abnormalities or other causes of embolic stroke are detected on routine monitoring. Extended cardiac monitoring may include the non-invasive cardiac monitor for 24 hours, 48 hours, or extended 30-day monitoring, as well as newer technology using an implantable cardiac rhythm device (Seet, Friedman, & Rabinstein, 2011). The use of extended monitoring techniques in the early period following stroke has helped identify patients with occult or undetected atrial fibrillation.

Therapeutic cardioversion and anti-arrythmics for rhythm control have not been shown to reduce stroke risk (Wyse et al., 2002). Anticoagulation is effective in prevention of stroke, and close medical monitoring is recommended for stroke prevention in patients with atrial fibrillation (Hart, Pearce, & Aguilar, 2010). For patients with mechanical prosthetic cardiac valves, warfarin is recommended with a target INR 3.0 for prevention of embolic stroke (Furie et al., 2011). Bio-prosthetic heart valves are not considered to be a significant risk factor for an embolic ischemic stroke, and unless cardiac imaging suggests otherwise, aspirin is typically prescribed.

The forms of anticoagulation to prevent ischemic vary depending on the presence of a stroke and the stability after ischemic stroke. Short-term anticoagulation can be accomplished with IV heparin or weight-based SQ low molecular weight heparinoids (LMWH). These agents are often used in the initial stages after stroke, when initially introducing anticoagulant agents and when bridging is necessary while anticoagulation must be interrupted. The benefit of short-term anticoagulation in acute stroke patients is that the effects can be easily reversible and it has a shorter half-life.

Long-term anticoagulation to reduce the risk of stroke may be accomplished by the use of daily oral Warfarin or Dabigatran. Warfarin dosing and response must be monitored with serum analysis to achieve target INR values. Dabigatran is a newer anticoagulant agent that works as a direct thrombin inhibition; it was approved recently, after the RE-LY trial demonstrated safety and efficacy compared to Warfarin. Dabigatran is an orally dosed medication administered twice daily, and no serum monitoring is required for dosing. Dosage adjustments are necessary in patients with renal impairment (Connolly et al., 2009).

Aspirin use for primary stroke prevention in the setting of atrial fibrillation is not well supported in the medical literature. It may be used as an alternative option in patients who are deemed high risk and when anticoagulation therapy cannot be safely administered (Furie et al., 2011).

Thrombotic stroke prevention
Antiplatelet therapy
Primary prevention with aspirin is recommended for prophylaxis of cardiovascular events, including stroke, in persons who are at high risk when the benefits outweigh the risks associated with treatment. The high-risk patient, by definition, is a person who has a 6–10% risk of ischemic stroke within 10 years (Furie et al., 2011). Aspirin is also recommended for primary stroke prevention in women who are considered high risk (age 65 or older with controlled blood

pressure), but aspirin is not recommended for prevention of first stroke in low-risk individuals.

Secondary prevention with aspirin

It is well documented in the stroke literature that aspirin therapy prevents recurrent stroke in patients with recent TIA or strokes of non-embolic etiology. The dosage range is wide and spans from 50 mg/day–1500 mg/day, although the most commonly used doses are 81 mg or 325 mg daily. The mechanism of aspirin therapy is that it irreversibly affects platelet function by decreasing the platelet aggregation. This in turn leads to a reduction in the potential for thrombosis and prolonged bleeding time (Antithrombotic Trialists C., 2002). The well-recognized potential risks of aspirin therapy include bleeding and gastrointestinal upset/hemorrhage.

Dipyridimole combined with aspirin is an oral agent that is approved for secondary stroke prevention in non-cardioembolic stroke. Dipyridimole acts by inhibiting phosphodiesterase and supplements prostacyclin-related platelet aggregation inhibition. Recommended dosing is twice daily, which provides 25 mg aspirin and 200 mg dipyridimole per dose (Diener et al., 1996). The most commonly reported side effects are headache and gastrointestinal upset.

Clopidogrel is a platelet receptor antagonist that is also an approved therapy for secondary stroke prevention. It is dosed once daily at 75 mg and has a similar safety profile to aspirin alone (CAPRIE Steering Committee, 1996). A potential medication interaction exists with medications that are metabolized via the CYP2C14 hepatic track. Proton pump inhibitors are included in this category and have been shown to reduce effectiveness of clopidogrel. Consideration of alternate medication agents for the treatment of heartburn or gastroesophageal reflux is recommended. Clopidogrel is an acceptable alternative in patients who have an aspirin allergy.

The co-administration of clopidogrel and aspirin has not been shown to reduce recurrent stroke, but does increase the risk of major hemorrhage (Diener et al., 2004). The only current recommendation for combination antiplatelet therapy with aspirin and clopidogrel is in patients who have undergone carotid stenting (Bhatt et al., 2001). The combined effects of these two antiplatelet agents are beneficial in reducing stent thrombosis, and therapy is generally continued for 3 months post-stenting. Following this initial period and after carotid ultrasound is performed to validate stent patency, single antiplatelet therapy is most often prescribed.

Ticlodipine is an additional antiplatelet agent that was approved for secondary prevention of ischemic stroke. It has similar effects on platelet aggregation to clopidogrel. The recommended dosing is 250 mg twice daily. The side-effect profile has resulted in limited clinical use. These potential side effects include severe neutropenia, thrombotic thrombocytopenic purpura (TTP), aplastic anemia, gastrointestinal upset, and rash. In patients who are initially prescribed ticlodipine, complete blood count monitoring every 2 weeks is recommended to monitor for the hematologic adverse effects (Drug Information Online, 2011). Clinically its use is reserved for patients who are intolerant or allergic to aspirin or who have failed aspirin therapy.

RISK FACTOR MODIFICATION
Carotid stenosis

For carotid stenosis, the medical literature supports intervention to revascularize the cerebral circulation when carotid atherosclerotic plaque measures 70% stenosis and there is evidence of active neurologic sequel referable to that vascular territory. A recently completed CREST trial compared carotid endaterectomy to carotid artery stenting in patients with 70% carotid stenosis and a clinical stroke or TIA in the appropriate vascular territory. It reported no difference in mortality or morbidity in terms of myocardial infarction or recurrent stroke rates between the two interventional groups (Brott et al., 2010). This trial exclusively examined the treatment in patients with symptomatic carotid stenosis. Symptomatic stenosis is defined as a clinical symptom consistent with a TIA, non-disabling stroke, or transient monocular blindness confirmed by diagnostic arterial testing that reveals ipsilateral stenosis of the internal carotid artery. For the patient with less severe degrees of carotid stenosis, there may be an indication for revascularization, but this recommendation is highly dependent on the medical co-morbidities and the presence of stenosis or occlusion in the contralateral carotid artery. In the case of less than 50% carotid stenosis, there is no data to support revascularization. In the asymptomatic patient, a more in-depth clinical evaluation is necessary to warrant intervention.

Hypertension – In a recent statement by the AHA detailing primary prevention of stroke, regular blood pressure screening is recommended and medication therapy is indicated when the SBP exceeds 140 mm HG or DBP exceeds 90 mm HG. The JNC7 recommendations divide hypertension into three categories: prehypertensive, Stage 1 hypertension, and Stage 2 hypertension (Chobanian et al., 2003). In patients with prehypertension (defined as SBP 120–139 mm Hg or DBP 80–89 mm Hg), regular monitoring and education on health-promoting lifestyle modifications to reduce the possible of progression to stage 1 or 2 hypertension and prevention of cardiovascular disease is recommended. These lifestyle changes include weight reduction, dietary approaches to stop hypertension (DASH), dietary sodium restriction, aerobic physical exercise, and moderate alcohol intake. Stage 1 hypertension is defined as SBP 140–159 mm HG or DBP 90–99 mm HG, and Stage 2 hypertension is defined as SBP >160 mm Hg or DBP > 100 mm Hg. In both stage 1 and stage 2 hypertension, medication therapy is recommended in addition to lifestyle modifications and regular monitoring. JNC7 recommendations also recognize that most patients will require two antihypertensive medications to achieve desired blood pressure goals (Chobanian et al., 2003). When hypertension coexists with diabetes, there is evidence that more aggressive blood pressure lowering is effective in reducing the risk of ischemic stroke (Furie et al., 2011).

Hyperlipidemia – Elevations in serum cholesterol and its components are directly related to increased risk of vascular disease. This is true not only for coronary artery disease, but ischemic stroke as well. Prescribing medications in the Statin group is effective, in addition to diet, weight management, and physical activity, in reducing both total cholesterol and low-density lipoprotein cholesterol (LDL-C). Current recommendations for the LDL-C level in patients with TIA or ischemic stroke and evidence of atherosclerosis are directed to achieve and maintain LDL-C less than 100 mg/dl (Furie et al., 2011). The SPARCL trial was specifically designed to evaluate the benefit of cholesterol lowering in stroke patients without evidence of CHD. The results showed that by introducing atorvastatin, patients who accomplish a more than 50% reduction in LDL-C reduce their stroke risk by approximately 35%

(Amarenco et al., 2007). This information, coupled with evidence demonstrating the lowering of Triglyceride levels (Freiberg et al., 2008) and increasing high-density lipoprotein cholesterol (HDL-C) (Sanossian et al., 2007), suggests that maintaining all three common lipid levels is important for the prevention of stroke and TIA.

Diabetes – It is estimated that nearly 8% of the adult population in the United States have diabetes mellitus (American Diabetes Association, 2010). Diabetes results in elevated serum glucose that occurs when insufficient or ineffective insulin excretion fails to counteract carbohydrate intake. Diabetes increases the risk of first stroke, but with appropriate identification and effective glucose management, recurrent stroke incidence can be reduced. Current recommendations for primary prevention of stroke in patients with diabetes are coupled with those of hypertension and hyperlipidemia. The patient who is diabetic is likely to also have additional risk factors for stroke, including hypertension and hyperlipidemia, which should be aggressively co-managed.

Cigarette smoking is a well-recognized risk for ischemic stroke. The most widely accepted mechanism is twofold. Acute effects appear to increase thrombus formation in arteries with evidence of atherosclerosis, and chronic smoking contributes to progression of atherosclerosis in general (Burns, 2003). Education and resources directed at smoking cessation are essential for patients and their families with stroke and TIA. This education should be provided during the acute phase of treatment, and resources for ongoing smoking cessation efforts should be included for the post-discharge phase.

Diet/nutrition/exercise – Sedentary lifestyle and obesity have been strongly associated with many of the known risk factors for stroke. Hypertension, diabetes, and hyperlipidemia have been discussed in detail above and can further be impacted by improvements in diet and physical activity. The guidelines for the primary prevention of stroke recommend the following:

- Reduction in sodium intake to lower blood pressure
- Increased intake of potassium to lower blood pressure
- DASH (Dietary Approaches to Stop Hypertension) style diet
- A diet rich in fruits and vegetables to lower the risk of stroke

- Increased physical activity to lower the risk of stroke
- Adults should engage in 150 minutes/week of moderate-intensity exercise or
- 75 minutes/week of vigorous physical activity
- Weight reduction is recommended to lower blood pressure and reduce the risk of stroke
- (Guidelines for the primary prevention of stroke 2010)

ACUTE CARE
Thrombolytics

With improved recognition by the general public, the establishment of protocols for pre-hospital personnel, and better prepared emergency departments (ED), the treatment of acute ischemic stroke patients continues to improve. IV t-PA was the first therapy to be approved for acute ischemic stroke in 1996 after the completion of the NIH-sponsored NINDS trial. Since that time, the role of the nurse in assessing and providing high-level care for acute stroke patients has been stressed in both protocol development and educational efforts.

On arrival to the ED, the identification of the patient with a potential stroke should prompt the collection of several important data points including time the patient was last known to be normal neurologically, detailed neurologic exam or NIHSS (see Table 3.2), serum glucose, past medical history, and current medications. Prioritization of diagnostic testing to obtain a non-contrasted CT scan of the brain and laboratory assessment of glucose and CBC are needed to exclude potential contraindications/risks for the use of IV thrombolytic therapy. A multidisciplinary approach by ED physicians, nurses, and neurologist is needed to determine the eligibility of patients who meet the criteria for IV t-PA and to deliver therapy within 3 hours of known symptom onset. The development and use of protocols that streamline the process are commonly seen and yield more consistent screening and treatment. Table 3.3 lists inclusion and exclusion criteria that are used to determine the patients' eligibility for IV t-PA administration.

The nurse is a vital member of the team in the assessment and administration of treatment. Many ED nurses develop and maintain

Table 3.2 NIHSS Scoring

1a. **Level of Consciousness** (LOC) – is the patient alert, drowsy, etc.
0 = Alert
1 = Drowsy
2 = Stuporous
3 = Coma

1b. **LOC Questions** – ask the patient the month and their age
0 = answers both correctly
1 = answers one correctly
2 = both incorrect

1c. **LOC Commands** – ask the patient to open/close eyes and the grip/release non-paretic hand
0 = obeys both correctly
1 = obeys one correctly
2 = both incorrect

2. **Best gaze** – horizontal – with eyes open – patient follows finger or face
0 = normal
1 = partial gaze palsy
2 = forced deviation of the eyes

3. **Visual** – test by confrontation – introduce visual stimulus to upper/lower field quadrants
0 = no visual loss
1 = partial hemianopia
2 = complete hemianopia
3 = bilateral hemianopia

4. **Facial Palsy** – ask patient to smile/show teeth, raise eyebrows, and squeeze eyes shut
0 = normal
1 = minor
2 = partial
3 = complete

5. **Motor arm** – extend arms to 90 degrees and score drift/movement
0 = no drift
1 = drift
2 = can't resist gravity
3 = no effort against gravity
4 = no movement (amputation or joint fusion – untestable – explain)

6. **Motor Leg** – elevate leg to 30 degrees and flex at hip. Always tested supine. Test legs individually
0 = no drift
1 = drift
2 = can't resist gravity
3 = no effort against gravity
4 – no movement (amputation or joint fusion – untestable - explain)

(*Continued*)

Table 3.2 (*Continued*)

7. **Limb Ataxia** – finger-to-nose, heel-to-shin tests performed on both sides
0 = absent
1 = present in one limb
2 = present in two limbs

8. **Sensory** – use pinprick to test face, arm, leg, trunk – compare side to side. Assess awareness of being touched
0 = normal
1 = partial loss
2 = severe loss

9. **Best Language** – as patients to name objects, describe picture, read a sentence
0 = no aphasia
1 = mild to moderate aphasia
2 = severe aphasia
3 = mute

10. **Dysarthria** – evaluate speech clarity by asking patient to repeat words
0 = normal articulation
1 = mild to moderate dysarthria
2 = near to unintelligible
If intubated or other barrier – untestable – explain

11. **Extinction/Inattention** – use info from prior testing to determines neglect or double simultaneous stimuli testing
0 = no neglect
1 = partial neglect
3 = complete neglect

Source: http://www.ninds.nih.gov/doctors/NIH_stroke_scale.pdf. Courtesy of the National Insitutes of Health National Institute of Neurological Disorders and Stroke.

competency in the mixing and dose calculation for IV t-PA and for the NIHSS assessment. Once the decision to treat is established, vigilant nursing care is necessary to monitor the patient for complications during IV thrombolytic administration and for the ensuing 24-hour period after therapy is delivered to monitor for potential adverse events. Vital signs monitoring (blood pressure, pulse, SaO_2, and respiratory rate) and monitoring of the neurologic examination is frequent: every 15 minutes during the 1-hour infusion and for the first hour after the infusion is complete, then every 30 minutes for the next 6 hours, then hourly until the initial 24-hour period is complete. If any neurologic exam worsening is noted, the nurse should notify the physician responsible for the patients care and prepare for repeat CT imaging to rule out intracerebral hemorrhage

Table 3.3 Inclusion/Exclusion Criteria for IV thrombolytics[45]

Inclusion criteria
Onset of symptoms less than 3 hours before beginning treatment
Neurologic presentation consistent with ischemic stroke
Baseline CT scan negative for intracranial hemorrhage

Exclusion criteria
Evidence of intracranial hemorrhage by CT or suspicion of subarachnoid hemorrhage
Recent intracranial or intraspinal surgery, serious head trauma, or stroke in previous 3 months

Intracranial neoplasm, arteriovenous malformation, or aneurysm
History of intracranial hemorrhage
Uncontrolled hypertension at the time of treatment (SBP > 185 mmHg or DBP > 110 mm Hg)

Active internal bleeding
INR > 1.7
Use of IV heparin within the preceding 48 hours with an elevated a PTT
Platelet count of < 100,000/mm3
Patients with major or early infarct signs on CT
Glucose < 50 or > 400 mg/dL

Table created from information found in Adams, H. P., Jr., del Zoppo, G., Alberts, M. J., et al. (2007). Guidelines for the early management of adults with ischemic stroke: A guideline from the American Heart Association/American Stroke Association Stroke Council, Clinical Cardiology Council, Cardiovascular Radiology and Intervention Council, and the Atherosclerotic Peripheral Vascular Disease and Quality of Care Outcomes in Research Interdisciplinary Working Groups: The American Academy of Neurology affirms the value of this guideline as an educational tool for neurologists. [Erratum appears in *Stroke 2007 38*(9), e96], [Erratum appears in Stroke *2007 38*(6),e38]. *Stroke, 38*(5),1655–1711.

or swelling. Strict blood pressure parameters are established and should be followed to avoid hypertension that can increase the risk of hemorrhage (see Table 3.4).

Admission to an intensive care unit (ICU) with specialty nursing care is necessary following the administration of IV t-PA. Nurses should be trained in the NIHSS and be knowledgeable about potential complications for patients who have received IV thrombolytic therapy. The use of standard order sets and protocols is encouraged to reinforce the frequency of monitoring and assessment and to set parameters for blood pressure range, blood pressure treatment, and general care of the patient.

Table 3.4 Blood pressure management in the setting of IV thrombolytics[39]

Pre-treatment

If SBP > 185 mmHg or DBP > 110 mmHg, consider treatment with:

- Labetalol IV 10-20 mg over 1–2 minutes – may repeat one time
- Nitropaste topical 1–2 inches
- Nicardipine infusion – start infusion at 5 mg/hour then titrate up to 15 mg/hour as needed with increases of 2.5 mg every 5–15 minutes

If blood pressure is not reduced to desired levels, then do not administer IV t-PA.

Post-treatment

Monitor BP every 15 minutes during the 60-minute infusion of IV t-PA

- then every 15 minutes for 1 hour after infusion is completed
- then every 30 minutes for 6 hours
- then hourly until 24 hours post-initial infusion

Blood pressure goals SBP < 185 mmHg and DBP > 110 mmHg

If BP exceeds goals, consider treatment with:

- Labetalol 10 mg IV over 1–2 minutes – may be repeated every 10-20 min to maximum dose of 300 mg
- Labetalol infusion of 2–8 mg/min
- Nicardipine infusion – start 5 mg/min and titrate up to max dose of 15 mg/hr
- Nipride infusion should be considered only if blood pressure cannot be controlled with nicardipine or labetalol.

Adapted from *Stroke 2009 40*, 2911–2944, table 10, p. 2920. Comprehensive overview of nursing and interdisciplinary care of the acute ischemic stroke patient. A scientific statement from the American Heart Association. Printed with permission from Wolters Kluwer Health.

Interventional treatment

Advances in neuroimaging have allowed stroke neurologists to better understand vascular occlusion and plan for intervention. Although IV t-PA is the only approved medication for acute ischemic stroke, the field of vascular interventional neurology has continued to advance to delineate the role of intra-arterial therapy. Intra-arterial therapy includes both the pharmacologic use of thrombolytic agents delivered via catheter angiography to the site of vessel occlusion, and the use of mechanical clot retrieval devices to relieve an arterial occlusion and restore blood flow to the brain. Currently, at many established stroke centers, the assessment of arterial status is accomplished in the acute phase either by CTA or MRA of the extracranial and intracranial cerebral circulation. When a patient is found to have occlusion of a large artery (middle cerebral, carotid, vertebral, or basilar artery), consideration for interventional treatment is discussed. The concomitant availability of cerebral perfusion imaging by both computed tomography perfusion (CTP) and magnetic resonance perfusion (MRP) is often used to assess the viability of the brain tissue supplied by an occluded vessel. These imaging techniques help guide the practitioner to distinguish between an already infarcted brain (or the ischemic core) and tissue at risk (or penumbral brain tissue). All of this requires the availability of a radiologist, neurologist, and interventionally trained specialist to review and incorporate the data obtained from these additional diagnostic evaluations.

There are currently two mechanical clot retrieval devices that are FDA approved for use in acute ischemic stroke to accomplish vessel recanalization. The Merci retrieval device was approved after the completion of the MERCI trial in 2005 (Smith et al., 2005). This device is deployed through a base catheter to the site of the arterial occlusion and utilizes a corkscrew-type tip with filamentous strands to help retrieve the clot. The Penumbra device was approved based on the results of the Penumbra trial that was released in 2008 (Bose et al., 2008). The Penumbra device uses external suction and a macerating catheter that is used to penetrate the clot. The goal is to break the clot into smaller pieces and then apply suction to remove the clot from the artery lumen. Both of these devices have an extended time window for use that can span up to 8 hours after the onset of stroke symptoms. These interventional approaches are indicated when patients do not qualify for IV t-PA or fail to have vessel recanalization after IV t-PA administration. Following any neurointerventional procedure, the stroke patient should also be cared for in an ICU setting with highly skilled nurses capable of performing the NIHSS assessment, close hemodynamic monitoring, and management, guided by a post-procedure-specific order set or protocol.

Nursing care
Efforts to maintain cerebral perfusion to limit brain tissue ischemia are the primary goal in the acute period after ischemic stroke. Neurologic recovery may be seen in the early stages after stroke when the ischemic brain tissue is reperfused prior to tissue infarction

occurring. Close monitoring and specialty nursing care delivered in stroke units have been shown to improve outcomes in stroke patients. Patients who have received IV thrombolysis or intra-arterial intervention should be admitted to an ICU where continuous cardiac monitoring, detailed neurologic examinations, and high-level nursing care can be provided. Additionally, patients who experience large strokes, without intervention or thrombolytics, who are at risk for neurologic or hemodynamic decline should be cared for in a critical care environment where the expertise of the physician and nurses can best assess and manage the patient in a tenuous state.

Acute care
The primary principles of acute care for the stroke patients do not differ from other critically ill patients. Assessment and management of the ABC's is the priority. Airway protection and patency is vital to ensure adequate oxygenation. Breathing pattern assessments including rate, regularity, and depth also contribute to oxygenation and are measures by respiratory rate and SaO_2 values. Circulation is supported by both heart rate and blood pressure. Monitoring for variations in pulse rate that range from bradycardia to rapid ventricular rates in the setting of atrial fibrillation is essential. Blood pressure goals and therapy to manage BP must be individualized depending on the use of thrombolytics, results of diagnostic testing including status of vessel patency, volume, and location of stroke, and the patients' medical co-morbidities.

Support of hemodynamic stability
Neurologic
The principles of management following stroke are aimed at supporting cerebral perfusion while balancing the potential for edema generation and the risk of worsening ischemia, as well as the risk of hemorrhagic transformation. As detailed earlier in this chapter, ischemic stroke results from arterial occlusion that prevents oxygen and glucose delivery to neuronal cells. The use of IV thrombolytic therapy and neurointerventional therapy is directed at re-establishing cerebral blood flow. Research studies have shown that when vessel recanalization occurs, patients often have an improvement in neurologic exam measured by the NIHSS and better

outcomes are associated with early clinical neurologic improvements (Kharitonova et al., 2011). Regular standardized neurologic monitoring by trained nurses and documentation of variations is necessary to detect and document changes in the neurologic examination.

Increased intracranial pressure may result if the stroke is large with respect to the amount of tissue involved and swelling occurs, or if hemorrhage occurs following stroke. Swelling or cerebral edema occurs commonly in the setting of large strokes that may involve more than one lobe of the brain. It is also more common to see swelling in young stroke patients and those with large cerebellar strokes with limited space to accommodate for swelling. Intracerebral hemorrhage is a known risk associated with the use of IV thrombolytics and interventional approaches to therapy. In the original NINDS trial, 6.4% of the patients treated with IV t-PA developed a hemorrhage that resulted in a deterioration of the neurologic exam. This is referred to as a symptomatic hemorrhage because there is a change in the neurologic status associated with the hemorrhage. Asymptomatic hemorrhages occur when there is evidence of blood on the repeat imaging but no associated neurologic change is noted. These can be described as hemorrhagic transformation, or petechial hemorrhage within the stroke tissue. Urgent repeat brain imaging is required if there is neurologic worsening clinically and should be performed at 24 hours on all patients regardless of neurologic status. This urgent and 24-hour CT or MRI will help identify the size and location of stroke and rule out edema and hemorrhage.

Clinically, the most common early symptoms of increased intracranial pressure (ICP) either from edema or hemorrhage include: patient complaints of headache, decline in motor function, decline in level of consciousness, nausea, agitation, and alterations in respiratory pattern, pulse or BP. Later signs of increased ICP include changes in pupil reaction to light and difficulty in arousing the patient, and can progress to instability in airway protection, pulse, and BP.

Cerebral perfusion can also be augmented by the use of appropriate positioning of the patient. To maximize cerebral perfusion, nurses caring for the stroke patient should maintained the head of the bed at 30-degree elevation and try to maintain midline head and body positioning to prevent impediments to venous drainage. Blood pressure management is also essential and should be individualized to find the best balance to minimize the risk of hemorrhage and maintain adequate cerebral perfusion.

Respiratory

In the vast majority of ischemic stroke patients, respiratory compromise is not a common presenting clinical feature. It may be seen in patients with posterior circulation strokes that involve the pons or medulla, when lower cranial nerve involvement can lead to inadequate airway protection. In general, patients with anterior circulation strokes are maintain adequate respiratory rate and SaO_2 levels. Supplemental oxygen is recommended to maintain an SaO_2 of more than 92% in the acute stroke setting and can be administered via nasal cannula. Continuous monitoring of the respiratory rate and oxygen saturation is needed to detect inadequate airway protection. Many patients are at risk for aspiration pneumonia due to impaired swallowing and inadequate handling of oral secretions. Elevation of the head of the bed at 30 degrees is recommended to reduce the risk of aspiration and airway obstruction. Protocols for bedside dysphagia screening are necessary, and patients should be kept in a nothing-by-mouth (NPO) regime until safety in swallowing is documented.

Cardiac

The status of arterial vessel patency, presence of collateral flow, and use of thrombolytics or interventional therapy are used to determine goals for BP that influence cerebral perfusion.

IV thrombolytics – following IV t-PA, there is well-established literature to support close BP monitoring and use antihypertensive agents to maintain SBP < 185 mm Hg, DBP < 110 mm Hg for the first 24 hours following therapy (see Table 3.4) (Group TNIoNDaSr-PSS, 1995). The rationale for these tight parameters is to reduce the risk of hemorrhage following IV thrombolytic therapy. When two successive readings exceed the established parameters, either before, during, or within the 24-hour period following therapy, IV PRN agents or IV continuous infusion of antihypertensives are indicated. In the patient who has not received treatment with IV thrombolytics or interventional therapy, in general the BP parameters are liberalized to maximize cerebral perfusion pressure and encourage flow through collaterals. The generally accepted guidelines include no urgent treatment or use of IV PRN agents unless the SBP > 220 mm Hg or DBP > 120 mm Hg in the acute stroke patient without evidence of end organ damage or other complications associated with the stroke (Summers et al., 2009).

- Interventional therapy – goals for BP management are individualized for interventionally treated patients depending in the therapy provided, the size of the stroke, and status of vessel patency. In general, when patient receives any treatment that may increase the risk of hemorrhagic conversion, BP is controlled in ranges similar to those used in the IV thrombolytic therapy population (see Table 3.4).
- Vessel patency – The treatment and success of therapy to relieve vessel occlusions are varied. The goals for BP management are dependent on this information coupled with the size of the stroke. In general, if cerebral arteries remain occluded, the blood pressure is liberalized to enhance collateral flow and alternative means of maintaining cerebral perfusion are employed. The primary goal of liberalizing blood pressure is to improve flow to the penumbra, or tissue that may be receiving marginal flow around the stroke core.
- Intravenous access is necessary in the acute phase of ischemic stroke to deliver fluids and medications. In the patient who is being considered for IV thrombolytic treatment, two peripheral lines are recommended so that concomitant PRN medications can be administered without disruption of thrombolytics. The choice of IV fluids solutions is also important and dextrose-containing solutions are avoided in the setting of stroke. Normal saline solution (NSS) is routinely ordered to maintain hydration and avoid hypotension.
- In the situation where the patient is hypotensive and neurologic fluctuations occur in the setting of lower blood pressure values, vasopressors may be considered to maintain higher BP to support cerebral perfusion. Generally, this therapy is avoided in patients who have been treated with IV thrombolytics or who have received interventional therapy. One clinical situation that

may warrant the use of vasopressors includes the patient with carotid occlusion who is relying on cerebral perfusion via collaterals that is BP or position dependent. In this setting, clinical changes in the neurologic exam including worsening of limb weakness or speech are observed when the head of the patient's bed is elevated or the BP falls. The use of vasopressors to raise the BP is temporary and may be continued for a short time while autoregulation or revascularization occurs.

Glucose management – Hypoglycemia should be ruled on initial assessment by EMS or emergency room personnel. If the serum glucose is below 60, correction is recommended to rule out hypoglycemia as the etiology of stroke like symptomatology. Repeat assessment of the neurological status should occur after correction of low serum glucose. If a clinical deficit continues to be present, consideration for treatment should proceed as it would in a patient with normoglycemia.

Hyperglycemia or elevated serum glucose is also known to worsen outcome in patients with acute ischemic stroke (Bae et al., 2005). Strict protocols to control serum glucose in the acute phase following stroke is needed and the use of insulin infusions is often necessary to achieve target values. Many institutions use insulin protocols to guide the management of hyperglycemia and reduce the risk of over correction. This monitoring and treatment requires attentive nursing care. Scientific statements regarding the use of IV thrombolytics also include precautionary recommendations for patients with severely elevated glucose in the acute phase of strokes. Poor outcomes including increased mortality, increases size of stroke, and increased risk of hemorrhagic transformation may result (Summers et al., 2009).

Temperature management – Fever in the setting of acute cerebral ischemia may result in clinical worsening and expansion of infracted brain tissue volume. Several theories to explain this relationship have been discussed in the literature, and temperature elevations likely increase the metabolic demands of the cerebral tissue. In an already stressed or underperfused situation, the concomitant presence of fever may result in less blood flow to vulnerable penumbral tissue (Summers et al., 2009). Therapies to maintain normothermia in the acute situation include topical cooling, central cooling by indwelling catheter, or medication therapy with acetaminophen. Frequent assessment of temperature is necessary to maintain normal body temperature.

Other nursing support and prevention

Gastrointestinal – Efforts to provide oral fluids, medications, and nutrition to patients should be initiated only after careful evaluation to determine safety of swallowing. Dysphagia is a common finding in this patient population and can result in aspiration pneumonia if patients are not carefully assessed to determine safe mechanics of swallowing. Many stroke centers follow a defined protocol for screening and early introduction of medication and fluid. A formal evaluation by a speech and language pathologist is recommended to further delineate the need for modifications in consistency of foods and the need for additional precautions to prevent aspiration.

If a patient is unable to safely swallow within the first 24–48 hours, consideration for inserting a nasogastric enteral feeding tube and initiation of enteral nutrition is indicated to avoid nutritional depletion. In the short term, enteral nutrition through a temporary nasogastric tube is often used to provide sufficient caloric intake and hydration for the patient who is unable to swallow safely. If more long-term enteric nutrition or hydration is needed, the insertion of a Percutaneous Endoscopic Gastrostomy (PEG) tube may be needed. Malnourishment is very common in stroke patients and is associated with higher complication rates and poor outcomes (Summers et al., 2009).

Integumentary – Due to impaired mobility and sensation, impaired bowel and bladder control, and often the use of thrombolytics, stroke patients are at higher risk of alterations in skin integrity and the potential for breakdown. Routine skin care and inspection by nursing professionals have improved over the past decade, and most hospitals target assessment and prevention of skin breakdown on all levels of nursing care. The stroke patient is at increased risk and requires routine inspection, turning, and repositioning to reduce this risk. When IV thrombolytics are used, there is an increased risk of bleeding and bruising that can be seen at IV sites, venapuncture, and to vulnerable tissue, which may be evident on the skin superficially. Automatic BP cuffs used during the acute period for frequent monitoring notoriously result in extensive bruising of the upper arm, and are thus discouraged. The inability of patients to turn themselves or reposition off pressure points also places the stroke patient at higher risk for skin breakdown. The most common points where pressure and breakdown occur are the posterior aspect of the heals, coccyx, elbows, and back of the head. Repositioning and assessment are necessary to identify areas at risk and implement strategies to limit disruptions to skin integrity. An additional risk is present in patients with impaired sensory perception. In this situation, the patient may not receive triggers or input in the form of pain to indicate that a skin area is at risk for injury.

Musculoskeletal – The patient who is diagnosed with an ischemic stroke frequently has some degree of muscle weakness or paralysis. Depending on the size of the tissue involved and location within the brain, this can vary from mild weakness or incoordination to flaccid or spastic paralysis. In either situation, care in positioning, movement, and transfers should be directed at preserving the range of motion in the affected limb, preventing atrophy, and preventing falls. When the patient is determined to be hemodynamically and neurologically stable, attempts to mobilize them are initiated by nursing, physical therapy, and occupational therapy. These early mobility actions include sitting at the side of the bed, transfer to sit out of the bed in a chair, and, when possible, standing at the bedside and ambulation with assistance. All initial attempts to get out of bed or ambulate should be performed with the assistance of a member of the health care team to document safety and stability. Consultations for physical and occupational therapy are common and should be included to determine the need for post-hospital rehabilitation.

Deep vein thrombosis (DVT) and pulmonary emboli (PE) are recognized complications from immobility, and prevention strategies should be implemented in this high-risk population of patients. If the stroke patient is unable to ambulate independently within 48 hours of admission to the hospital, DVT prophylaxis should be ordered and administered. Acceptable forms of DVT prophylaxis include the use of compression stocking and pneumatic compression devices, SQ heparin, LMWH, or the use of systemic heparin for stroke prevention when indicated. Nursing care should include assessment of DVT risk and documentation of the use of DVT prophylaxis in the daily progress notes.

LONG-TERM CARE OF THE STROKE PATIENT
Maintaining adequate cerebral perfusion

Blood pressure management – Hypertension is a documented risk factor for both ischemic and hemorrhagic stroke and should be monitored and treated to achieve target values. The use of antihypertensives is common following ischemic stroke. After the acute phase of care when vessel patency and the size and location of the stroke burden are determined, introduction of oral medications is recommended to treat elevated BP. Several classes of agents are used and treatment should be selected based on the patients' previous medications, renal function, and medical co-morbidities. The oral agents that may be ordered include beta blockers, calcium channel blockers, angiotensin converting enzyme (ACE) inhibitors, and angiotensin receptor blockers (ARB). These antihypertensives may also be combined with diuretic agents to improve BP control. There are also centrally acting alpha-blocking agents that are used in situations where BP control is difficult to achieve with the agents listed above. Stroke patients with diagnosed or suspected hypertension should be instructed to routinely monitor their BP following discharge, either through home monitors or in a physicians' offices, and to create and maintain a log of readings for review at a subsequent physician visit to best determine BP trends and averages.

If a patient has neurological decline or fluctuation following initiation antihypertensive therapy, consideration for allowing the BP to remain slightly higher may be indicated. A thorough evaluation of the status of the large arteries both intracranially and extracranially should be performed, if not already done, to determine if there is a flow-limiting stenosis or vessel occlusion. In this setting, BP reduction may worsen tissue ischemia when the cerebral blood flow is dependent on higher BP values.

Lipid management – Hyperlipidemia is a well-documented risk factor for ischemic stroke. An assessment of serum-fasting lipid values should be ordered during the acute hospitalization. If the LDL-C is >100 mg/dl or T cholesterol is > 200 mg/dl, treatment is necessary. Recommendations for dietary and lifestyle modifications should be provided in addition to the discharge instruction, and oral statin therapy has been approved for secondary stroke prevention in individuals with stroke or TIA. Repeat analysis of fasting lipid panel and liver function testing are necessary to monitor for response to therapy with statins and to assess for side effects. This repeat laboratory assessment should be ordered within 6–8 weeks of initiation of therapy. The patients should also be instructed to notify a physician if they develop muscle pain or muscle weakness following stroke when a statin medication is ordered. Adjustments to therapy should be made to achieve target LDL-C and total cholesterol.

Maximizing function – rehab concepts

There is strong evidence that an organized plan that includes interdisciplinary stroke rehabilitation reduces not only mortality, but also the likelihood of stroke survivors requiring institutional care and long-term disability. This organized approach to care in the post-stroke period also enhances recovery and allows patients increased independence with activities of daily living (Kalra & Langhorne, 2007). The evaluation of patients for post-hospital rehabilitation is an essential link in the chain of stroke recovery and usually occurs after the patient is medically stable and prior to discharge.

In the stroke literature, there are several concepts that may be used to rehabilitate the stroke patient. Each person and concept for rehabilitation must be individually considered based on the patient's functional and clinical deficits and goals for recovery. The general goal of inpatient acute rehabilitation is to facilitate return of the stroke patient to community-based living. The general goal of outpatient and home therapy is to maximize recovery to allow independent living.

Rehabilitation is provided by physical, occupational, and speech/language therapists. Initially, they assess the strength, endurance, range of motion, gait (when possible), and sensory deficits of the stroke patient to determine the best course of rehabilitation therapy. In general, physical therapy is directed at practicing muscle movement in the impaired limb in a repetitive manner to encourage brain plasticity. "Neuroplasticity" is a term that refers to the ability of the brain and nervous system to change structurally and functionally as a result of input from the environment (Shaw & McEachern, 2001). In the stroke setting, aggressive rehabilitative therapy serves as the environmental stimulus to encourage new pathways of communication in the brain that can lead to functional physical improvement. The goals of rehabilitation following stroke are to encourage neuroplasticity that results in improved function and outcomes for stroke survivors.

Constraint induced therapy has been studied in a variety of trials and is used in patients with upper extremity deficits to stimulate motor recovery. The unaffected hand is tethering or mitted, preventing use, so that the paretic hand and arm are forced to function. It should be noted that the baseline level of motor function necessary for this type of therapy included intact wrist extension and finger and arm movement. Constraint induced therapy is conducted for several hours per day in a concentrated manner 5–6 days a week for a short period of time (2–6 weeks), and has been shown to improve upper extremity function of the affected limb (Page, Levine, & Leonard, 2005).

Robot-assisted therapy can also be used in the patient with upper or lower extremity weakness from stroke. The device is applied to the extremity and is programmed to help accomplish movement when the patient initiates movement. The devices can offer resistance to movement to strengthen both flexors and extensor muscles. The concept of robot-assisted therapy is that practice with movement can improve motor function (Kahn et al., 2006).

POST-ACUTE-STROKE PLACEMENT AND CARE

Following stroke, an assessment of neurological deficits and their impact on the patients functioning is typically undertaken. This assessment is performed by members of the multidisciplinary health care team and includes speech-language therapy, physical therapy, occupational therapy, and often services of physicians from the physical medicine and rehabilitation specialty. The goal of this assessment is to determine if post-hospital rehabilitation therapy is indicated to maximize functional recovery. As stated earlier in this chapter, stroke is the leading cause of disability among adults, and all efforts to engage the stroke survivor in rehabilitation services that will restore independence and self-care are warranted.

The discharge planning begins soon after admission and involves not only the rehabilitation specialties listed above, but also the patient, family, social services, and nursing case management. Rehabilitation should be considered in all patients and arranged either in the inpatient or outpatient setting to maximize physical recovery from stroke.

1. Patients are considered for **discharge to home** when there are limited functional deficits from the ischemic stroke. These may include mild arm or face weakness, numbness, mild speech abnormalities, or mild visual disturbance. Depending on the severity of symptoms and availability of 24/7 supervision in the home environment, the care management team and rehabilitation professionals make a recommendation that best ensures that the patient can be safely cared for. A home assessment following discharge is often ordered either for home nursing or a specialty therapy (physical, occupational, speech/language), with follow-up therapy or monitoring as needed. In patients with no residual neurologic deficits, it is not unusual for them to be discharged to home with education/instructions on new medications, lab assessments that are needed, and instructions to follow up with their PCP in 1–2 weeks.

2. A stroke patient who has more significant neurological deficits and requires ongoing 24/7 nursing care is considered for **discharge to an acute inpatient rehabilitation** setting. The minimum criteria for admission to an inpatient rehabilitation facility are that the patient must be able to participate in a minimum of 3 hours of acute therapy services per day. State by state, the definition and licensing of rehabilitation beds and hospitals differs and, similarly, patients also have varying degrees of insurance coverage to provide for inpatient acute rehabilitation. This type of rehabilitation is considered when possible to assist the patient with retraining self-care and activities of daily living, safety in transfers, strengthening, mobility, and communication. Depending on the severity of the residual stroke deficits, several days to several weeks of therapy may be necessary before the patient can safely transition back into the home.

3. When a patient has more severe residual neurologic deficits or is medically not stable enough to participate in aggressive inpatient rehabilitation, **transfer to a skilled nursing level care** is often considered. While in this setting, the patient's condition can be monitored and managed with 24/7 nursing care while often receiving less intense rehabilitative services. Patients with

more severe stroke often require additional care to ensure that nutrition, skin integrity, and medical management of risk factors are optimized. Even though a patient may not be eligible for acute inpatient rehabilitation initially, reassessment by a physical medicine and rehabilitation specialist is often advised within 4–6 weeks post stroke to determine if the patient may qualify after he/she becomes medically more stable. If this is not possible, ongoing physical, occupational, and speech-language therapy should be continued with the goal of maximizing recovery and, if possible, transition to home.

Following stroke, medical care is commonly directed at risk factor management and prevention of recurrent stroke. These priorities are needed in addition to maximizing physical recovery through an organized plan of therapy. Recognition of the psychological effect of stroke and disability on both the patient and family also must be acknowledged and addressed. For many patients, stroke is sudden, unexpected, and results in changes that impact the remainder of their life. Depression and despair are common following stroke and can negatively impact the benefits of therapy. It is necessary for health care professionals at all levels who interface with stroke survivors and their families to assess mood, coping, and overall adaptation in all settings. Referrals to the patient's medical care provider, neurologist, social services, or a psychological care provider should be initiated if there is a concern noted.

SUMMARY
Acute therapy and medical care of the stroke patient has evolved over the past 15 years. Abundant research continues to be conducted to identify treatment and strategies to both prevent and maximize recovery following stroke.

REFERENCES
Adams, H. P., Jr., Bendixen, B. H., Kappelle, L. J., et al. (1993). Classification of subtype of acute ischemic stroke. Definitions for use in a multicenter clinical trial. TOAST. Trial of Org 10172 in Acute Stroke Treatment. *Stroke*, 24(1), 35–41.
Adams, H. P., Jr., del Zoppo, G., Alberts, M. J., et al. (2007). Guidelines for the early management of adults with ischemic stroke:

A guideline from the American Heart Association/American Stroke Association Stroke Council, Clinical Cardiology Council, Cardiovascular Radiology and Intervention Council, and the Atherosclerotic Peripheral Vascular Disease and Quality of Care Outcomes in Research Interdisciplinary Working Groups: The American Academy of Neurology affirms the value of this guideline as an educational tool for neurologists. [Erratum appears in *Stroke 2007 38*(9), e96], [Erratum appears in *Stroke 2007 38*(6), e38]. *Stroke, 38*(5), 1655–1711.

Albers, G. W., Amarenco, P., Easton, J. D., Sacco, R. L., & Teal, P. (2004). Antithrombotic and thrombolytic therapy for ischemic stroke: The Seventh ACCP Conference on Antithrombotic and Thrombolytic Therapy. *Chest, 126*(3 Suppl), S483–S512.

Alsheikh-Ali, A. A., Kitsios, G. D., Balk, E. M., Lau, J., & Ip, S. (2010). The vulnerable atherosclerotic plaque: Scope of the literature. *Annals of Internal Medicine, 153*(6), 387–395.

Amarenco, P., Goldstein, L. B., Szarek, M., et al. (2007). Effects of intense low-density lipoprotein cholesterol reduction in patients with stroke or transient ischemic attack: The Stroke Prevention by Aggressive Reduction in Cholesterol Levels (SPARCL) trial. *Stroke, 38*(12), 3198–3204.

American Diabetes Association. (2010). Standards of medical care in diabetes – 2010. [Erratum appears in *Diabetes Care 2010 33*(3), 692]. *Diabetes Care, 33*(Suppl 1), S11–S61.

American Heart Association (2010). CPR statistics. Available at: http://www.heart.org/HEARTORG/CPRAndECC/Whatis CPR/CPRFactsandStatistics_UCM_307542_Article.jsp (accessed April 26, 2010).

American Medical Association (2009). *Handbook of first aid and emergency care*. New York: Random House.

Antithrombotic Trialists C. (2002). Collaborative meta-analysis of randomised trials of antiplatelet therapy for prevention of death, myocardial infarction, and stroke in high risk patients. [Erratum appears in *BMJ 2002 324*(7330), 141]. *BMJ, 324*(7329), 71–86.

Bae, H.-J., Yoon, D.-S., Lee, J., et al. (2005). In-hospital medical complications and long-term mortality after ischemic stroke. *Stroke, 36*(11), 2441–2445.

Bhatt, D. L., Kapadia, S. R., Bajzer, C. T., et al. (2001). Dual antiplatelet therapy with clopidogrel and aspirin after carotid artery stenting. *Journal of Invasive Cardiology*, *13*(12), 767–771.

Bose, A., Henkes, H., Alfke, K., et al. (2008). The Penumbra System: A mechanical device for the treatment of acute stroke due to thromboembolism. *American Journal of Neuroradiology*, *29*(7), 1409–1413.

Brott, T. G., Hobson II, R. W., Howard, G., et al. (2010). Stenting versus endarterectomy for treatment of carotid-artery stenosis. [Erratum appears in *New England Journal of Medicine 2010 363*(5), 498], [Erratum appears in *New England Journal of Medicine 2010 363*(2), 198]. *New England Journal of Medicine*, *363*(1), 11–23.

Burns, D. M. (2003). Epidemiology of smoking-induced cardiovascular disease. *Progress in Cardiovascular Diseases*, *46*(1), 11–29.

CAPRIE Steering Committee (1996). A randomised, blinded, trial of clopidogrel versus aspirin in patients at risk of ischaemic events (CAPRIE). *CAPRIE Steering Committee. Lancet*, *348*(9038), 1329–1339.

Chobanian, A. V., Bakris, G. L., Black, H. R., et al. (2003). The Seventh Report of the Joint National Committee on Prevention, Detection, Evaluation, and Treatment of High Blood Pressure: The JNC 7 report. [Erratum appears in *Journal of American Medical Association 2003 290*(2), 197]. *Journal of American Medical Association*, *289*(19), 2560–2572.

Connolly, S. J., Ezekowitz, M. D., Yusuf, S., et al. (2009). Dabigatran versus warfarin in patients with atrial fibrillation. [Erratum appears in *New England Journal of Medicine 2010 363*(19), 1877]. *New England Journal of Medicine*, *361*(12),1139–1151.

Diener, H.-C., Bogousslavsky, J., Brass, L. M., et al. (2004). Aspirin and clopidogrel compared with clopidogrel alone after recent ischaemic stroke or transient ischaemic attack in high-risk patients (MATCH): Randomised, double-blind, placebo-controlled trial. *Lancet*, *364*(9431), 331–337.

Diener, H. C., Cunha, L., Forbes, C., Sivenius, J., Smets, P., & Lowenthal, A. (1996). European Stroke Prevention Study 2: Dipyridamole and acetylsalicylic acid in the secondary prevention of stroke. *Journal of the Neurological Sciences*, *143*(1–2), 1–13.

Drug Information Online (2011). Ticlid. *Drugs.com*. Online at: http://www.drugs.com/pro/ticlid.html (accessed November 22).

Freiberg, J. J., Tybjaerg-Hansen, A., Jensen, J. S., & Nordestgaard, B. G. (2008). Nonfasting triglycerides and risk of ischemic stroke in the general population. *Journal of American Medical Association*, *300*(18), 2142–2152.

Furie, K. L., Kasner, S. E., Adams, R. J., et al. (2011). Guidelines for the prevention of stroke in patients with stroke or transient ischemic attack: A guideline for healthcare professionals from the American Heart Association/American Stroke Association. *Stroke*, *42*(1), 227–276.

Gage, B. F., Waterman, A. D., Shannon, W., Boechler, M., Rich, M. W., & Radford, M. J. (2001). Validation of clinical classification schemes for predicting stroke: Results from the National Registry of Atrial Fibrillation. *Journal of American Medical Association*, *285*(22), 2864–2870.

Goldstein, L. B., Bushnell, C. D., Adams, R. J., et al. (2011). Guidelines for the primary prevention of stroke: A guideline for healthcare professionals from the American Heart Association/American Stroke Association. [Erratum appears in *Stroke 2011 42*(2), e26]. *Stroke*, *42*(2), 517–584.

Group TNIoNDaSr-PSS. (1995). Tissue plasminogen activator for acute ischemic stroke. The National Institute of Neurological Disorders and Stroke rt-PA Stroke Study Group. *New England Journal of Medicine*, *333*(24), 1581–1587.

Hart, R. G., Pearce, L. A., & Aguilar, M. I. (2010). Meta-analysis: Antithrombotic therapy to prevent stroke in patients who have nonvalvular atrial fibrillation. *Annals of Internal Medicine*, *146*(12), 857–867.

Jones R. (2006). Asphyxia, strangulation. Available at: http://www.forensicmed.co.uk (accessed November 22, 2011).

Kahn, L. E., Lum, P. S., Rymer, W. Z., & Reinkensmeyer, D. J. (2006). Robot-assisted movement training for the stroke-impaired arm: Does it matter what the robot does? *Journal of Rehabilitation Research & Development*, *43*(5), 619–630.

Kalra, L., & Langhorne, P. (2007). Facilitating recovery: Evidence for organized stroke care. *Journal of Rehabilitation Medicine*, *39*(2), 97–102.

Kannel, W. B., & Benjamin, E. J. (2008). Status of the epidemiology of atrial fibrillation. *Medical Clinics of North America*, *92*(1), 17–40.

Kharitonova, T., Mikulik, R., Roine, R. O., et al. (2011). Association of Early National Institutes of Health Stroke Scale improvement with vessel recanalization and functional outcome after intravenous thrombolysis in ischemic stroke. *Stroke*, *42*(6), 1638–1643.

Lunetta, P., & Modell, J. H. (2005). *Forensic pathology reviews*. Vol 3. Totowa, NJ: Humana Press.

Ng, K. W. P., Loh, P. K., & Sharma, V. K. (2011). Role of investigating thrombophilic disorders in young stroke. *Stroke Research and Treatment*. Article ID 670138. 9 pages.

Page, S. J., Levine, P., & Leonard, A. C. (2005). Modified constraint-induced therapy in acute stroke: A randomized controlled pilot study. *Neurorehabilitation & Neural Repair*, *19*(1), 27–32.

Prockop, L. D., & Chichkova, R. I. (2007). Carbon monoxide intoxication: An updated review. *Journal of the Neurological Sciences*, *262*(1–2), 122–130.

Reininger, A. J., Bernlochner, I., Penz, S. M., et al. (2010). A 2-step mechanism of arterial thrombus formation induced by human atherosclerotic plaques. *Journal of the American College of Cardiology*, *55*(11), 1147–1158.

Sanossian, N., Saver, J. L., Navab, M., & Ovbiagele, B. (2007). High-density lipoprotein cholesterol: An emerging target for stroke treatment. *Stroke*, *38*(3), 1104–1109.

Seet, R. C. S., Friedman, P. A., & Rabinstein, A. A. (2011). Prolonged rhythm monitoring for the detection of occult paroxysmal atrial fibrillation in ischemic stroke of unknown cause. *Circulation*, *124*(4), 477–486.

Shaw, C. A., & McEachern, J. C. (2001). *Toward a theory of neuroplasticity*. Philadelphia: Psychology Press.

Smith, W. S., Sung, G., Starkman, S., et al. (2005). Safety and efficacy of mechanical embolectomy in acute ischemic stroke: Results of the MERCI trial. *Stroke*, *36*(7), 1432–1438.

Summers, D., Leonard, A., Wentworth, D., et al. (2009). Comprehensive overview of nursing and interdisciplinary care of the acute ischemic stroke patient: A scientific statement from the American Heart Association. *Stroke*, *40*(8), 2911–2944.

Welch, K. M. A., Caplan, L. R., Reis, D. J., Siesjo, B. K., & Weir, B. (eds.). (1997). *Primer on cerebrovascular diseases*. New York: Academic Press.

Writing Group M, Lloyd-Jones, D., Adams, R. J., et al. (2010). Heart disease and stroke statistics – 2010 update: A report from the American Heart Association. [Erratum appears in *Circulation, 2010 121*(12), e260. Note: Stafford, Randall [corrected to Roger, Veronique L.] *Circulation, 121*(7), e46–e215.

Wyse, D. G., Waldo, A. L., DiMarco, J. P., et al. (2002). A comparison of rate control and rhythm control in patients with atrial fibrillation. *New England Journal of Medicine, 347*(23),1825–1833.

Yenari, M., Kitagawa, K., Lyden, P., & Perez-Pinzon, M. (2008). Metabolic downregulation: A key to successful neuroprotection? *Stroke, 39*(10), 2910–2917.

Young, G. B. (2009). Clinical practice: Neurologic prognosis after cardiac arrest. *New England Journal of Medicine, 361*(6), 605–611.

Intracerebral Hemorrhage

4

Tarek Dakakni and Michael L. "Luke" James

Evidence-Based Nursing Care for Stroke and Neurovascular Conditions,
First Edition. Edited by Sheila A. Alexander.
© 2013 John Wiley & Sons, Inc. Published 2013 by John Wiley & Sons, Inc.

Intracerebral hemorrhage (ICH) is defined as bleeding into the parenchyma of the brain, usually originating from a small penetrating artery, to be distinguished from subarachnoid hemorrhage (SAH), which is a bleeding into the subarachnoid space originating from one of the main vessels of the Circle of Willis. The annual incidence of ICH in the United States is around 100,000 people and accounts for 10–15% of all strokes (Gebel & Broderick, 2000). However, this rate is expected to double in the next 50 years due to the increasing age of the population and the concomitant use of anticoagulation therapy for co-morbid cardiovascular disease. At present, the incidence of ICH varies based on age, race, and sex (Thom et al., 2006) and tends to double every decade of age after 35 years (Manno et al., 2005). Overall, ICH is more common in men than women, although this varies as age advances (Qureshi et al., 2001). Additionally, in the United States, minority populations such as African Americans, Asians, and Hispanics show a statistically higher predilection for ICH than Americans of European origin (Kissela et al., 2004; Labovitz et al., 2005).

RISK FACTORS

Several important risk factors with disease-modifying capacity exist in ICH. Hypertension is the single most important risk factor for spontaneous ICH, especially in people with poorly controlled hypertension and a history of noncompliance with antihypertensive medications (Qureshi et al., 2001). Second, anticoagulation with warfarin within the clinically relevant treatment range increases the risk of ICH to an absolute rate of nearly 1.8% per year. The annual risk of ICH with warfarin use is directly related to the degree to which a patient is anticoagulated (i.e., longer prothrombin times [PT] and international normalized ratios [INR] are associated with greater risk of ICH). Other predictors of anticoagulant-related ICH are advanced patient age, history of ischemic stroke, and hypertension (Hart, Boop, & Anderson, 1995; Steiner, Rosand, & Diringer, 2006). Finally, alcohol consumption, tobacco use, and recreational drug abuse increases the risk of ICH (Mayer & Rincon, 2005). Among young men and women (younger than 50 years of age), modifiable independent risk factors for ICH include current cigarette smoking, consumption of two or more alcoholic drinks daily, and use of cocaine and/or amphetamine (Feldmann et al., 2005).

Finally, patients with cerebral amyloid angiopathy (CAA) are at increased risk of developing ICH. This clinical syndrome is typified by spontaneous lobar hemorrhages in elderly patients with cognitive decline and is discussed in further detail below. However, it is clear that ICH related to CAA demonstrates a greater propensity for recurrence but does not appear related to modifiable risk factors. Furthermore, evidence suggests that cerebral microbleeds may indicate a higher risk of future ICH and may be a marker of cerebral small-vessel disease and CAA (Labovitz et al., 2005; Koennecke, 2006).

MORTALITY AND PROGNOSIS

ICH has traditionally been associated with dismal morbidity and mortality as well as high societal costs. In the published literature, the 6-month mortality rate is between 30% and 50% (Qureshi et al., 2001; Manno et al., 2005) with only 20% of patients regaining functional independence at 6 months (Mayer & Rincon, 2005). Perhaps more astounding is the fact that ICH also results in substantial medical costs due to acute hospital and chronic care expenses with significant loss of productivity (Reed et al., 2001). An epidemiologic model of incidence, survival, and recurrence based on a review of the literature found that the lifetime cost per patient of a first ICH occurring in 1990 was estimated to be greater than $120,000, with an aggregate lifetime cost of approximately $6 billion in the United States alone. Interestingly, of the expense incurred in the first 2 years following a first ICH, in-hospital costs incurred accounted for 45% of the total costs, long-term ambulatory care accounted for 35%, and nursing home costs accounted for 17.5% (Taylor et al., 1996)

A number of prognostic models exist for determining outcome after ICH (Table 4.1). The most widely used and validated clinical tool is the ICH Score (Hemphill III et al., 2001) (see discussion that follows). It has repeatedly demonstrated nearly 80% correlation with outcomes out to 6 months after injury. However, although a number of prognostic factors have been validated, it should be noted that "withdrawal of care" orders initiated by a treating team have introduced significant bias in the traditional sense of

Table 4.1 The ICH score: (14)

ICH points			
GSC score:		IVH:	
13-15	0	Yes	1
5-12	1	No	0
3-4	2		
Age		Infratentorial location	
>80	1	Yes	1
<80	0	No	0
ICH volume		Total score	
>30 cm	1		
<30 cm	0		

30 day mortality - 0 points 0% mortality, 1 point 13% mortality, 2 points 26% mortality, 3 points 725 mortality, 4 points 97% mortality and 5 points 100% mortality.

Reprinted from Hemphill J. C., 3rd, Bonovich D. C., Besmertis L., et al. 2001, with permission from Wolters Kluwer Health.

prognosis, as the idea of patients expected to have a poor outcome leads to self-fulfilling prophecies (Becker et al., 2001). Furthermore, without distinguishing in the literature between patients that died despite maximal medical intervention and those that died after withdrawal of support, factors involved in actual long-term outcome cannot be fully evaluated. In fact, the most important prognostic variable in determining outcome after ICH is the level of medical support provided and the timing of initiation of Do Not Resuscitate (DNR) orders (Zahuranec et al., 2001). As an example, Zurasky et al. (2005) found that limitation or withdrawal of life-sustaining interventions was the most common cause of death (68%) after ICH in a review of over 1,400 subjects.

Though clinical variables, such as age and hematoma size, are consistently highly correlative with mortality, it is likely that biological signatures may augment existing tools. It is well established that genetic polymorphisms are implicated in prognosis, especially apolipoprotein E (ApoE) (Alberts et al., 1995; McCarron et al., 1995; McCarron et al., 2003; James, Blessing, Bennett et al., 2009). Genetic variants appear to influence pathophysiology after ICH through regulation of end protein products. Further, evolving evidence suggests a role for protein serum "biomarkers" as adjuncts to clinical prognostic tools to improve the clinician's ability to predict long-term outcome (James, Blessing, Phillips-Bute et al., 2009) and as a means to differentiate various causes of cerebral injury (Laskowitz et al., 2009). Finally, there is hope that these genetic and biologic signatures may lead to the development of targeted therapeutics (James, Sullivan, Lascola et al., 2009; James et al., 2010).

CLASSIFICATION

ICH can be divided into subtypes based on the etiology and generally distinguished through medical history, neurological examination, and imaging.

Hypertensive ICH

Also known as spontaneous or primary cerebral hemorrhage, hypertensive ICH is generally considered to be secondary to chronic hypertension resulting in degenerative changes, known as lipohyalinosis, in the small penetrating cerebral arterioles. This results in consistent locations for hypertensive ICH demonstrated by computed tomography (CT) imaging: basal ganglia, thalamus, pons, cerebellum, and lobar regions. Approximately 2% of hypertensive ICH occurs in multiple locations. In addition, hematoma formation can expand in the intraventricular cerebrospinal fluid (CSF) space and is termed intraventricular hemorrhage (IVH). About half of hypertensive ICH cases originate in the basal ganglia (resulting from rupture of the ascending lenticulostriate branches of the middle cerebral artery), a third in the cerebral hemispheres (penetrating cortical branches of the anterior, middle, or posterior cerebral arteries), and a sixth in the brainstem or cerebellum (penetrating branches of the posterior inferior, anterior inferior, or superior cerebellar arteries). ICH in the pons usually originates from paramedian branches of the basilar artery; hemorrhages in the thalamus usually originate from the ascending thalmogeniculate branches of the posterior cerebral artery (Qureshi et al., 2001; Mayer & Rincon, 2005). Generally, hypertensive ICH is dichotomized into supra- and infratentorial injuries based on the hematoma's relation to the tentorium. Infratentorial ICH is generally considered a surgical disease, as evacuation of these hematomas can result in excellent clinical outcomes and is considered standard of care. This is in stark contrast to supratentorial ICH (STICH), in which surgical evacuation

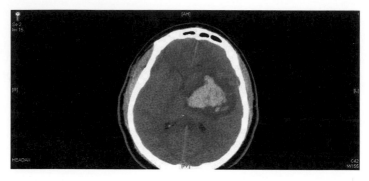

Fig. 4.1 Left Basal Ganglia Hypertensive ICH on CT imaging

appears to play a limited role at best. Finally, hypertensive ICH results in a robust inflammatory response occurring over the first 48 to 72 hours after initial hematoma formation, which may not be seen in other forms of ICH (Figure 4.1).

Lobar ICH
Generally occurring in the elderly, lobar ICH is secondary to amyloid deposition in the cerebral vasculature related to CAA. These hemorrhages are much more likely to demonstrate multiple foci and be associated with evidence of microhemorrhages on magnetic resonance imaging (MRI). Emerging evidence has implicated a strong association between Alzheimer's disease, amyloid angiopathy, and lobar ICH (Labovitz et al., 2005).

Anticoagulant therapy-induced ICH
Coagulopathy related to warfarin use is the second most common cause of ICH, accounting for 14% of all ICH. Being directly related to the degree of anticoagulation as demonstrated by the latency of the INR, the location of the bleed can occur anywhere within the brain parenchyma. Further, the degree to which the hematoma may expand over the first 24 hours after ICH is associated with the elevation of INR on presentation. In addition, neurological outcome is directly related to the rapidity with which anticoagulation is reversed (Aguilar et al., 2007).

ICH secondary to any primary hematologic disorder

An infrequent cause of ICH, hematologic diseases such as leukemia, aplastic anemia, or thrombocytopenia may involve ICH as a symptom. Systemic indications for these diseases are generally known prior to ICH or are evident on presentation. Treatment is related to addressing the primary disease (Quinones-Hinojosa et al., 2003).

Arteriovenous malformation (AVM)

An AVM consists of a tangle of dilated vessels that form an abnormal communication between the arterial and the venous systems in the brain. As a developmental abnormality, AVMs are usually seen in younger patients with history of headaches or seizures. A general rule of thumb sets the lifetime risk of hemorrhage from an AVM to 105 minus the patient's age (Mast et al., 1997). When hemorrhage occurs, blood may enter to the subarachnoid space, producing a picture very similar to the SAH caused by an aneurysm, but generally less severe. Imaging by MRI, CT, or conventional angiogram can distinguish hemorrhages due to AVM from other causes. Treatment for AVMs is usually surgical after stabilization and recovery of the brain from ICH (Figure 4.2) (Stapf et al., 2006).

Cavernous angioma

Cavernous angiomas are vascular malformation consisting of a cluster of thin-walled veins within the brain parenchyma. With about 10% of lesions being multiple, there is an apparent autosomal

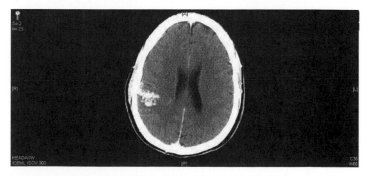

Fig. 4.2 ICH secondary to AVM on CT imaging

dominant inheritance pattern. Thus, not surprisingly, cavernous angiomas are more likely to be seen in younger patients with a history of seizure or headaches. In addition, there is a prototypical "popcorn" appearance on MRI due the presence of blood in different stages of resorption. Treatment is usually surgical (Washington, McCoy, & Zipfel, 2010).

Drug-use-associated ICH

Although excessive alcohol use is a risk factor for the development of ICH, the use of cocaine and/or amphetamine may be a primary cause of it. It is believed the use of these drugs results in increased blood pressure that then initiates hematoma formation. Chronic use of these drugs may result in damage to the cerebral arterioles, much like hypertension, which can then lead to ICH. Cocaine and amphetamine as a cause for ICH generally occur in a younger demographic than hypertensive ICH (Pozzi, Roccatagliata, & Sterzi, 2008).

Neoplasm

Glioblastoma multiforme is the most common primary brain tumor associated with ICH; however, the most common cause of ICH related to neoplasm is from metastatic malignancy to the brain, such as melanoma, lung, thyroid, renal, and choriocarcinoma. Lymphoma, especially associated with HIV/AIDS, is the second most common cause of primary brain tumor hemorrhage and has a typical ring-enhancing appearance on CT imaging (Figure 4.3). Finally, pituitary adenomas may rupture and extravasate blood in the suprasellar cistern, known as pituitary apoplexy.

Venous sinus thrombosis

ICH related to venous sinus thrombosis with cortical infarction is often related to a hypercoagulable state, pregnancy, and/or dehydration. The signature feature of isolated thrombosis of superficial cortical vein is the presence of large superficial hemorrhagic infarction. The diagnosis is made through MR venogram, and treatment consists of heparinization to prevent extension of the thrombosis (Bentley, Figueroa, & Vender, 2009).

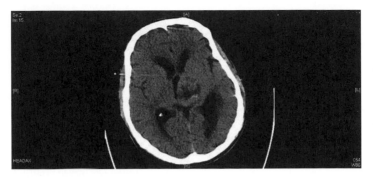

Fig. 4.3 Small ICH associated with a brain tumor with edema, midline shift, and hydrocephalus on CT imaging

Ischemic stroke with hemorrhagic conversion

Hemorrhagic conversion after an ischemic infarct is most common in large-vessel embolic strokes. In addition, the use of systemic tPA for the treatment of acute ischemic stroke carries a 6% risk of hemorrhagic conversion (The National Institute of Neurological Disorders and Stroke rt-PA Stroke Study Group, 1995).

Trauma

Diagnosed through history, traumatic ICH, or cerebral contusion, is often associated with other forms of intracranial hemorrhage, such as SAH and subdural hemorrhage (SDH). There may also be the presence of skull fractures and the classic coupe/contracoupe lesion on opposite poles of the brain. Cerebral contusions generally develop significant cerebral edema and may be associated with varying degrees of underlying axonal injury from traumatic brain injury (TBI) (Perel et al., 2010).

Mycotic aneurysm

Cerebral aneurysm may develop from embolic sources of infection, generally subacute bacterial endocarditis (SBE). This aneurysm can then rupture and result in ICH much like SAH. However, unlike ICH or SAH, treatment is through a prolonged course of antibiotics and clearing the primary infection (Kong & Chan, 1995).

Aneurismal subarachnoid hemorrhage

Aneurismal SAH from cerebral aneurysm rupture may have a primary intraparenchymal component and mimic hypertensive ICH. Differentiation occurs through imaging by CT or conventional angiogram.

DIAGNOSIS

Diagnosis of ICH is generally made through CT brain imaging in appropriately selected patients. Patients presenting with acute onset of localizing neurological symptoms should undergo emergent CT brain imaging. The presence of a hyperdense lesion on brain CT within the area of the brain that explains the patient's neurological symptoms should be considered ICH until proven otherwise. Further imaging by MRI or angiography may help provide a subtype diagnosis for the presence of ICH.

Brain CT also allows for an approximation of the hemorrhage volume, which is directly related to prognosis. This measurement is estimated by calculating the volume via AxBxC/2 method, where A is the longest axis of the hematoma, B is the perpendicular axis, and C is the number of cuts that show blood on CT (Gebel et al., 1998). Finally, CT angiogram or CT with contrast may be helpful in predicting the probability of hematoma expansion in the first 24 hours via the presence of the "spot sign," which is defined as any foci of enhancement within the hematoma (Delgado Almandoz, 2009).

CLINICAL MANIFESTATION

The clinical presentation varies depending on the location and the size of the hematoma (e.g., small hematomas might cause coma if they occur in the midbrain, whereas large hematomas may present with only a slight headache if located in the subcortical white matter). Furthermore, traditionally, ICH has been considered a monophasic event (hematoma formation). However, ICH is now understood as a dynamic and complex process that involves several distinct phases. Typically, ICH presents with a sudden onset of neurological deficit and impaired level of consciousness in the setting of high blood pressure. Traditionally, patients complain of headaches, nausea, and vomiting (especially if the hematoma occurs in the posterior fossa). In addition, seizures can be a common initial presentation of lobar ICH or ICH secondary to AVMs.

The degree of neurological deficit has the potential to worsen over the first 48 to 72 hours as the hematoma expands and cerebral edema is generated as a substantial amount of tissue damage occurs after an initial hemorrhage. The mechanisms that lead to early hematoma growth during the acute stage of ICH remain unclear, but a sudden increase in intracranial pressure (ICP), local tissue distortion and shear forces, and disruption of normal cerebral anatomy can lead to the enlargement of the hematoma with the addition of discrete hemorrhages at the periphery of the initial primary hematoma. Other changes that can contribute to early hematoma growth include vascular engorgement related to the reduction of venous outflow, early transient ischemia, and breakdown of the blood-brain barrier (Qureshi et al., 2001; Manno et al., 2005; Mayer & Rincon, 2005). Many hemorrhages continue to grow and expand several hours after symptom onset. Brott et al. (1997) reported that hematoma expanded in 26% of patients within 1 hour after the initial CT scan and in another 12% within 20 hours. A recent meta-analysis by Davis et al. (2006) that included patients with spontaneous ICH who underwent CT within 3 hours of onset and at 24-hour follow-up showed an even higher rate: 73% of patients exhibited some degree of hematoma growth over the first 24 hours and 38% had significant (>33%) expansion over this period (Kazui et al., 1996). Hematoma growth is an independent determinant of both mortality and functional outcome after ICH (National Institute of Neurological Disorders and Stroke Workshop, 2005). Predictors of hemorrhage expansion include initial hematoma volume, early presentation, irregular shape, liver disease, hypertension, hyperglycemia, alcohol use, and hypofibrinogenima (Fujii et al., 1998; Kazui et al., 1997).

As the initial hemorrhage and its expansion dissect along cerebral tissue planes, islands of intact neural tissue are encircled (Qureshi et al., 2001; Manno et al., 2005; Mayer & Rincon, 2005). Neurologic deterioration after this point is often attributed to the development of cerebral edema, which appears within hours secondary to clot retraction and extrusion of plasma proteins. Fluid begins to collect immediately in the region around the hematoma. Early edema around the hematoma results from the release and accumulation consists of osmotically active serum products from the clot. Plasma rich in thrombin and other coagulation end-products seeps into the surrounding brain tissue and is the primary trigger of the inflammatory process. Later, delayed thrombin formation may contribute directly to neuronal toxicity or indirectly through damage to the blood-brain barrier (Qureshi et al., 2001; Manno et al., 2005; Mayer & Rincon, 2005). Data suggest that ICH-induced inflammation represents a key factor leading to secondary brain damage (James, Warner, & Laskowitz, 2008; James, Sullivan, Lascola et al., 2009; James et al., 2010). Neuronal death in the region around the hematoma is predominately necrotic, with evidence implicating selected aspects of inflammatory response including the role of cytokines, transcription factor nuclear factor-kB, microglia activation, astrogliosis, and complement activation (Aronowski & Hall, 2009).

Further, the presence of IVH or cerebral edema evolving to occlude CSF drainage foramens can promote the occurrence of hydrocephalus. In the first few days after ICH, the most ominous complication is herniation due to progressive cerebral edema formation in the setting of large hemorrhage volume. In all cases, signs and symptoms of increased intracranial pressure (ICP) should be monitored, including decreased level of consciousness, impaired upward gaze, lethargy, vomiting, or a fixed dilated pupil. It is also common for systolic blood pressure to be elevated on presentation, especially in the setting of hypertensive or cocaine-induced ICH. Further, signs of chronic hypertension may be noticed, such as hypertrophic left ventricle on EKG.

Recurrence

The rate of recurrence of ICH depends largely on the etiology. Hypertensive hemorrhage is lowest at 2% per year if hypertension is adequately treated and patients remain compliant with the medication regimen. Lobar ICH related to CAA has an annual recurrence of approximately 10% and is largely not modifiable. Anticoagulant-associated ICH is directly related to the extent that the patient's INR is prolonged. The recurrence of ICH due to cocaine or amphetamine use is nearly zero if drug use is discontinued (Sansing et al., 2009).

MANAGEMENT

ICH is a medical emergency; early rapid diagnosis and management are important, especially since deterioration is common early after ICH onset. The following section is based largely on the most recent AHA/ASA recommendations from September 2010 (Morgenstern et al., 2010).

In the pre-hospital setting, any patient with neurologic symptoms suspicious for a stroke becomes the highest priority for rapid assessment and emergent transfer, as has been the case for suspected myocardial infarctions for decades. Immediate notification of the receiving facility prior to arrival will help coordinate the appropriate resources and personnel in order to streamline diagnosis and care. An important step is the incorporation of the regional emergency medical service (EMS) community into the continuum of stroke care along with the emergency department (ED) and the intensive care unit (ICU). This participation of the medical center, ICU, EMS, and ED staff in the educational activities and formal written agreements for triage to stroke centers is crucial to the success of these endeavors.

In the field, EMS providers must be prepared and able to follow the "ABCs" of resuscitation for all patients with signs of stroke, perform a pre-hospital stroke assessment, and alert the receiving facility as soon as possible. The patient's blood glucose should be checked, intravenous access established, and the last known well time should be determined. Timely transport is critical, but rapid transfer must be weighed against the benefits of triage to a stroke center with a stroke unit.

Upon arrival at the ED, all patients suspected of having an acute stroke should be triaged immediately to a high-priority area, and the following actions should be taken simultaneously: initiation of stabilization measures, assessment of vital signs, history and physical examination, a neurologic examination, diagnostics and imaging, and implementation of preventive strategies to minimize complications. An acute stroke pathway should be in place and activated, thus facilitating rapid diagnosis and resource utilization while minimizing delay to definitive diagnosis and therapy. General care includes assessment and support of the "ABCs" and evaluation of baseline vital signs. Blood pressure should be monitored closely with a determination regarding the treatment of hypertension. In addition, all hypoxemic patients should receive supplemental oxygen and the consideration for supplemental oxygen should be given to non-hypoxemic patients. Intravenous access should be established or confirmed, blood samples obtained for baseline laboratories (glucose, complete blood count, coagulation studies, platelets, electrolytes, cardiac enzymes, etc.), and 12-lead electrocardiogram obtained. The NIH Stroke Scale (NIHSS) should be assessed by ED staff to document baseline symptoms. Emergent CT scan of the brain is mandatory and should ideally be completed within 25 minutes of the patient's arrival in the ED, with immediate formal interpretation. If hemorrhage is noted on the CT scan, the acute stroke team should be consulted and consideration given for transfer to the ICU. In the setting of known ICH, any coagulopathy should be aggressively corrected, with the initiation of therapy immediately after verification of ICH. Finally, in semi-comatose patient (generally defined as a Glasgow Coma Score [GCS] of less than 9), consideration should be given for emergent neurosurgical consultation for extraventricular drainage (EVD) of CSF and ICP monitoring, especially in the setting of a CT demonstrating a large hematoma, significant cerebral edema, IVH, and/or hydrocephalus. Reversal of coagulopathy or placement of ICP monitor, if needed, should not wait for transfer to the ICU and should be initiated emergently in the ED.

Upon transfer to the ICU, the "ABCs" should be reassessed and supported as necessary. If an EVD has not been placed in the ED and the patient remains or has progressed to a semi-comatose state (GCS <9), emergent neurosurgical consultation should occur. Direct handover from ED nursing staff to ICU nursing staff should occur. Adequate intravenous access should be assessed, and initial examination should be made with the incorporation of the NIHSS. Involvement of the acute stroke team should be verified and the patient placed on the appropriate acute stroke clinical care pathway.

Vital signs should be closely monitored and the neurological exam repeated at frequent intervals, generally every hour or every other hour. In patients presenting with an elevated systolic blood pressure (BP) of greater than 160 mm Hg, lowering of systolic BP to 140 through intermittent or continuous intravenous administration of antihypertensive medications should be considered. If an ICP monitor is in place, cerebral perfusion pressure (CPP) of greater than 60 should also be incorporated as a target. A correlation exists between elevated BP and hematoma expansion in the first 24 hours after ICH, but this expansion can be attenuated in selected patients by acute lowering of the blood pressure (Anderson et al., 2010).

Patients with ICH in the setting of a coagulation factor deficiency or thrombocytopenia (less than 100 K platelets on complete blood count) should receive appropriate factor replacement therapy or platelets transfusion, respectively, although there is limited data to verify efficacy. Patients with an elevated INR secondary to oral anticoagulant use should have their coagulopathy reversed through cessation of warfarin administration, intravenous administration of Vitamin K, and administration of therapy to replace vitamin K-dependent factors through transfusion of either fresh frozen plasma (FFP) and/or prothrombin complex concentrate (PCC). PCC has not been shown to improve the long-term outcome compared to FFP, but reduced the amount of fluid volume the patient receives; it also contains fewer nonessential proteins for reversal of "warfarinization." Thus it is considered a reasonable alternative to FFP. Finally, consideration should be given to the administration of recombinant Factor VIIa (FVII) in the setting of ICH with a highly elevated INR (greater than 3). Though FVII does not replace other clotting factors beside Factor VII, its administration can quickly correct elevated INR to normal values and has proven efficacy in limiting hematoma expansion. However, routine use of FVII in all patients with ICH is not warranted as data do not support its efficacy (Mayer et al., 2008). The benefits of FVII are the rapidity of INR normalization and the low volume of fluid required to achieve this goal. However, using FVII is not recommended in ICH with normal INR secondary to the increasing risk of thromboembolic phenomenon. Finally, the utility of platelet transfusion in patients with ICH and a history of antiplatelet therapy is unclear and is considered investigational (Ducruet et al., 2010).

Frequent monitoring of serum glucose should occur and maintenance of normoglycemia is recommended. However, limited data suggest the efficacy of strict normoglycemic protocols in patients with ICH, despite excellent evidence that hyperglycemia worsens outcome (Godoy, Di Napoli, & Rabinstein, 2010).

At 24 hours after the initial hematoma formation, consideration should be given to repeat CT imaging to document the stabilization of hematoma expansion and the degree of cerebral edema. In addition, angiogram or CT angiogram may be useful to evaluate other etiologies of ICH other than induced hypertension. Finally, if hematoma expansion has occurred, it is reasonable to repeat imaging at 6- to 12-hour intervals until stabilization of the hemorrhage volume occurs.

ICH patients are at high risk for developing deep vein thrombosis (DVT) and pulmonary embolism because of limb paresis and prolonged immobilization. Dynamic compression stockings should be placed on admission. Within 48 hours after documentation of hematoma stabilization, administration of low-dose subcutaneous low-molecular-weight heparin or unfractioned heparin may be considered to prevent DVT.

Clinical seizures should be treated with antiepileptic medications, but the routine use of prophylactic anticonvulsants should not be performed. Risk of seizure increases in hematomas located near the cortex, and prophylaxis against seizure may be reasonable in these patients. Continuous EEG monitoring should be obtained after ICH in any patient with depressed mental status out of proportion to the degree of brain injury.

The usefulness of surgery for most patients with ICH is uncertain. Despite lack of definitive data, it is the standard of care for patients with cerebellar hemorrhage who are neurologically deteriorating due to brainstem compression and/or hydrocephalus to undergo surgical removal of the hemorrhage as soon as possible. Recent results from a multicenter randomized controlled clinical trial demonstrated that for patients presenting with lobar clot >30 ml and within 1 cm of the cortical surface, hematoma evacuation through open craniotomy may have some long-term benefit. However, the same trial demonstrated no efficacy for surgery applied to all individuals with supratentorial ICH (Mendelow et al., 2005).

A number of other issues in the medical management patients with intracerebral hemorrhage (ICH) remain to be resolved and/or adopted. Aggressive care in the early stages after ICH onset and postponement of new DNR orders until at least the second hospitalization day are recommended. Second, corticosteroids should be avoided, as randomized trials have failed to demonstrate their efficacy in patients with an ICH. Also, fever after ICH is common, particularly after IVH. Sustained fever after ICH is independently associated with poor outcome. Acetaminophen may be used without reservation in patients without hepatic disease. Induced normothermia via intravascular or surface cooling devices has been recommended in ICH patients for fever control, although evidence for the efficacy of these interventions in patients with neurologic disorders is meager (Badjatia, 2009).

Rehabilitation should begin as soon as is technically feasible. The extent of rehabilitation activities will depend on the patient's condition, but range-of-motion exercises can begin almost immediately in the ICU, even in comatose patients. It is reasonable that all patients with ICH have access to multidisciplinary rehabilitation, and those able to tolerate the acute rehabilitation environment should be transferred to such facilities as soon as possible.

REFERENCES

Alberts, M. J., Graffagnino, C., McClenny, C., et al. (1995). ApoE genotype and survival from intracerebral haemorrhage. *Lancet*, *346*(8974), 575.

Aguilar, M. I., Hart, R. G., Kase, C. S., et al. (2007). Treatment of warfarin-associated intracerebral hemorrhage: Literature review and expert opinion. *Mayo Clinic Procedures*, *82*(1), 82–92.

Anderson, C. S., Huang, Y., Arima, H., et al. (2010). Effects of early intensive blood pressure-lowering treatment on the growth of hematoma and perihematomal edema in acute intracerebral hemorrhage: The Intensive Blood Pressure Reduction in Acute Cerebral Haemorrhage Trial (INTERACT). *Stroke*, *41*(2), 307–312.

Aronowski, J., & Hall, C. E. (2005). New horizons for primary intracerebral hemorrhage treatment: Experience from preclinical studies. *Neurological Research*, *27*(3), 268–279.

Badjatia, N. (2009). Hyperthermia and fever control in brain injury. *Critical Care Medicine*, *37*(7 Suppl): S250–S257.

Becker, K. J., Baxter, A. B., Cohen, W. A., et al. (2001). Withdrawal of support in intracerebral hemorrhage may lead to self-fulfilling prophecies. *Neurology*, *56*(6), 766–772.

Bentley, J. N., Figueroa, R. E., & Vender, J. R. (2009). From presentation to follow-up: diagnosis and treatment of cerebral venous thrombosis. *Neurosurgical Focus*, *27*(5), E4.

Brott, T., Broderick, J., Kothari, R., et al. (1997). Early hemorrhage growth in patients with intracerebral hemorrhage. *Stroke*, *28*(1), 1–5.

Davis, S. M., Broderick, J., Hennerici, M., et al. (2006). Hematoma growth is a determinant of mortality and poor outcome after intracerebral hemorrhage. *Neurology*, *66*(8), 1175–1181.

Delgado Almandoz, J. E., Yoo, A. J., Stone, M. J., et al. (2009). Systematic characterization of the computed tomography angiography spot sign in primary intracerebral hemorrhage identifies patients at highest risk for hematoma expansion: the spot sign score. *Stroke*, *40*(9), 2994–3000.

Ducruet, A. F., Hickman, Z. L., Zacharia, B. E., et al. (2010). Impact of platelet transfusion on hematoma expansion in patients receiving antiplatelet agents before intracerebral hemorrhage. *Neurological Research*, *32*(7), 706–710.

Feldmann, E., Broderick, J. P., Kernan, W. N., et al. (2005). Major risk factors for intracerebral hemorrhage in the young are modifiable. *Stroke*, *36*(9), 1881–1885.

Fujii, Y., Takeuchi, S., Sasaki, O., et al. (1998). Multivariate analysis of predictors of hematoma enlargement in spontaneous intracerebral hemorrhage. *Stroke*, *29*(6), 1160–1166.

Gebel, J. M., & Broderick, J. P. (2000). Intracerebral hemorrhage. *Neurology Clinician*, *18*(2), 419–438.

Gebel, J. M., Sila, C. A., Sloan, M. A., et al. (1998). Comparison of the ABC/2 estimation technique to computer-assisted volumetric analysis of intraparenchymal and subdural hematomas complicating the GUSTO-1 trial. *Stroke*, *29*(9), 1799–1801.

Godoy, D. A., Di Napoli, M., & Rabinstein, A. A. (2010). Treating hyperglycemia in neurocritical patients: Benefits and perils. *Neurocritical Care*, *13*(3), 425–438.

Hart, R. G., Boop, B. S., & Anderson, D. C. (1995). Oral anticoagulants and intracranial hemorrhage: Facts and hypotheses. *Stroke*, *26*(8), 1471–1477.

Hemphill III, J. C., Bonovich, D. C., Besmertis. L., et al. (2001). The ICH score: A simple, reliable grading scale for intracerebral hemorrhage. *Stroke*, *32*(4), 891–897.

James, M. L., Blessing, R., Bennett, E., et al. (2009). Apolipoprotein E modifies neurological outcome by affecting cerebral edema but not hematoma size after intracerebral hemorrhage in humans. *Journal of Stroke & Cerebrovascular Disease, 18*(2), 144–149.

James, M. L., Blessing, R., Phillips-Bute, B. G., et al. (2009). S100B and brain natriuretic peptide predict functional neurological outcome after intracerebral haemorrhage. *Biomarkers, 14*(6), 388–394.

James, M. L., Sullivan, P. M., Lascola, C. D., et al. (2009). Pharmacogenomic effects of apolipoprotein e on intracerebral hemorrhage. *Stroke, 40*(2), 632–639.

James, M. L., Wang, H., Venkatraman, T., et al. (2010). Brain natriuretic peptide improves long-term functional recovery after acute CNS injury in mice. *Journal of Neurotrauma, 27*(1), 217–228.

James, M. L., Warner, D. S., & Laskowitz, D. T. (2008). Preclinical models of intracerebral hemorrhage: A translational perspective. *Neurocritical Care, 9*(1), 139–152.

Kazui, S., Minematsu, K., Yamamoto, H., et al. (1997). Predisposing factors to enlargement of spontaneous intracerebral hematoma. *Stroke, 28*(12), 2370–2375.

Kazui, S., Naritomi, H., Yamamoto, H., et al. (1996). Enlargement of spontaneous intracerebral hemorrhage: Incidence and time course. *Stroke, 27*(10), 1783–1787.

Kissela, B., Schneider, A., Kleindorfer, D., et al. (2004). Stroke in a biracial population: The excess burden of stroke among blacks. *Stroke, 35*(2), 426–431.

Koennecke, H. C. (2006). Cerebral microbleeds on MRI: Prevalence, associations, and potential clinical implications. *Neurology, 66*(2), 165–171.

Kong, K. H., & Chan, K. F. (1995). Ruptured intracranial mycotic aneurysm: A rare cause of intracranial hemorrhage. *Archives of Physical & Medical Rehabilitation, 76*(3), 287–289.

Labovitz, D. L., Halim, A., Boden-Albala, B., et al. (2005). The incidence of deep and lobar intracerebral hemorrhage in whites, blacks, and Hispanics. *Neurology, 65*(4), 518–522.

Laskowitz, D. T., Kasner, S. E., Saver, J., et al. (2009). Clinical usefulness of a biomarker-based diagnostic test for acute stroke: the Biomarker Rapid Assessment in Ischemic Injury (BRAIN) study. *Stroke, 40*(1), 77–85.

Manno, E. M., Atkinson, J. L., Fulgham, J. R., et al. (2005). Emerging medical and surgical management strategies in the evaluation and treatment of intracerebral hemorrhage. *Mayo Clinic Procedures, 80*(3), 420–433.

Mast, H., Young, W. L., Koennecke, H. C., et al. (1997). Risk of spontaneous haemorrhage after diagnosis of cerebral arteriovenous malformation. *Lancet, 350*(9084), 1065–1068.

Mayer, S. A., Brun, N. C., Begtrup, K., et al. (2008). Efficacy and safety of recombinant activated factor VII for acute intracerebral hemorrhage. *New England Journal of Medicine, 358*(20), 2127–2137.

Mayer, S. A., & Rincon, F. (2005). Treatment of intracerebral haemorrhage. *Lancet Neurology, 4*(10), 662–672.

McCarron, M. O., Hoffmann, K. L., DeLong, D. M., et al. (1995). Intracerebral hemorrhage outcome: Apolipoprotein E genotype, hematoma, and edema volumes. *Neurology, 53*(9), 2176–2179.

McCarron, M. O., Weir, C. J., Muir, K. W., et al. (2003). Effect of apolipoprotein E genotype on in-hospital mortality following intracerebral haemorrhage. *Acta Neurologica Scandinavica, 107*(2), 106–109.

Mendelow, A. D., Gregson, B. A., Fernandes, H. M., et al. (2005). Early surgery versus initial conservative treatment in patients with spontaneous supratentorial intracerebral haematomas in the International Surgical Trial in Intracerebral Haemorrhage (STICH): A randomised trial. *Lancet, 365*(9457), 387–397.

Morgenstern, L. B., Hemphill III, J. C., Anderson, C., et al. (2010). Guidelines for the management of spontaneous intracerebral hemorrhage: a guideline for healthcare professionals from the American Heart Association/American Stroke Association. *Stroke, 41*(9), 2108–2129.

National Institute of Neurological Disorders and Stroke Workshop (2005). Priorities for clinical research in intracerebral hemorrhage: A report. *Stroke, 36*(3), e23–e41.

Perel, P., Roberts, I., Shakur, H., et al. (2010). Haemostatic drugs for traumatic brain injury. *Cochrane Database Systemic Review, 2010*(1), CD007877.

Pozzi, M., Roccatagliata, D., & Sterzi, R. (2008). Drug abuse and intracranial hemorrhage. *Neurological Science, 29*(Suppl 2), S269–S270.

Quinones-Hinojosa, A., Gulati, M., Singh, V., et al. (2003). Spontaneous intracerebral hemorrhage due to coagulation disorders. *Neurosurgical Focus*, *15*(4), E3.

Qureshi, A. I., Tuhrim, S., Broderick, J. P., et al. (2001). Spontaneous intracerebral hemorrhage. *New England Journal of Medicine*, *344*(19), 1450–1460.

Reed, S. D., Blough, D. K., Meyer, K., et al. (2001). Inpatient costs, length of stay, and mortality for cerebrovascular events in community hospitals. *Neurology*, *57*(2), 305–314.

Sansing, L. H., Messe, S. R., Cucchiara, B. L., et al. (2009). Prior antiplatelet use does not affect hemorrhage growth or outcome after ICH. *Neurology*, *72*(16), 1397–1402.

Stapf, C., Mast, H., Sciacca, R. R., et al. (2006). Predictors of hemorrhage in patients with untreated brain arteriovenous malformation. *Neurology*, *66*(9), 1350–1355.

Steiner, T., Rosand, J., & Diringer, M. (2006). Intracerebral hemorrhage associated with oral anticoagulant therapy: Current practices and unresolved questions. *Stroke*, *37*(1), 256–262.

Taylor, T. N., Davis, P. H., Torner, J. C., et al. (1996). Lifetime cost of stroke in the United States. *Stroke*, *27*(9), 1459–1466.

The National Institute of Neurological Disorders and Stroke rt-PA Stroke Study Group. (1995). Tissue plasminogen activator for acute ischemic stroke. *New England Journal of Medicine*, *333*(24), 1581–1587.

Thom, T., Haase, N., Rosamond, W., et al. (2006). Heart disease and stroke statistics – 2006 update: A report from the American Heart Association Statistics Committee and Stroke Statistics Subcommittee. *Circulation, 113*(6), e85–e151.

Washington, C. W., McCoy, K. E., & Zipfel, G. J. (2010). Update on the natural history of cavernous malformations and factors predicting aggressive clinical presentation. *Neurosurgical Focus*, *29*(3), E7.

Zahuranec, D. B., Morgenstern, L. B., Sanchez, B. N., et al. (2001). Do-not-resuscitate orders and predictive models after intracerebral hemorrhage. *Neurology*, *75*(7), 626–633.

Zurasky, J. A., Aiyagari, V., Zazulia, A. R., et al. (2005). Early mortality following spontaneous intracerebral hemorrhage. *Neurology*, *64*(4), 725–727.

Subarachnoid Hemorrhage

5

Sheila A. Alexander

Evidence-Based Nursing Care for Stroke and Neurovascular Conditions,
First Edition. Edited by Sheila A. Alexander.
© 2013 John Wiley & Sons, Inc. Published 2013 by John Wiley & Sons, Inc.

Subarachnoid hemorrhage (SAH) is an emergent condition occurring when blood enters the space between the arachnoid and the pia. The blood mixes with the cerebrospinal fluid and bathes the exterior of the major cerebral blood vessels. It occurs in approximately 35,000 Americans each year. The most common cause of subarachnoid hemorrhage is due to rupture of a cerebral aneurysm occurring in 85% of patients with subarachnoid hemorrhage. Subarachnoid hemorrhage can also occur after rupture/leaking of an arteriovenous malformation (AVM) or due to trauma. In a small percentage of the population suffering subarachnoid hemorrhage, the cause of the bleeding is never found. Individuals on blood thinners or with clotting disorders are at increased risk of subarachnoid hemorrhage. Subarachnoid hemorrhage due to ruptured aneurysm or AVM occurs more often in females and Blacks. Risk of aneurysm rupture increases with age, with the average age of rupture being around 55 years old. Risk of AVM rupture most often occurs in the third decade of life. Subarachnoid hemorrhage after trauma is common, occurs more often in men than women, and occurs in all races and at all ages, although trauma is more common in the third, fourth, seventh, and eighth decade of life.

PATHOPHYSIOLOGY

Formation of cerebral aneurysms and AVMs is not well understood. AVMs appear to be purely congenital. Cerebral aneurysms often occur more frequently in family members of patients with aneurysms. Increased pressure in the vasculature puts undue strain on the weakened vessel walls of cerebral aneurysms and AVMs. The increased pressure overcomes the vessel walls' ability to contain it and the vessel ruptures, leaking blood out of the vasculature. When blood leaves the vasculature into the subarachnoid space, multiple problems occur. The initial increase in volume within the cranial vault leads to increased intracranial pressure. It is estimated that about 30% of people suffering subarachnoid hemorrhage do not survive the initial hemorrhage. For those surviving the initial bleed, additional problems are common. Blood exposed to the exterior surface of the major blood vessels supplying blood to the brain causes irritation and alterations in blood flow. Cerebral vasospasm is a common secondary event after subarachnoid hemorrhage, occurring when the blood vessels enter a transient, spastic state. During periods of spasm, the vessel constricts and the internal lumen becomes narrower, decreasing blood delivery to the tissue beyond that section of the blood vessel. For many patients, no symptoms present and full recovery can be expected. For 30% of patients experiencing subarachnoid hemorrhage, the decrease in blood delivery leads to hypoxia and/or ischemia to the tissue, termed delayed cerebral ischemia (DCI). Signs and symptoms of cerebral vasospasm and DCI are directly related to the area of brain tissue that is suffering from inadequate blood flow.

In 10–15% of patients recovering from subarachnoid hemorrhage (Claasen et al., 2002), cerebral edema develops due to alterations in the blood brain barrier, electrolyte imbalance, and/or fluid shifting into brain tissue.

In about 10% of patients recovering from aneurysmal subarachnoid hemorrhage, a second bleed due to re-rupture of the aneurysm will occur (Fujii et al., 1996; Molyneux et al., 2005). The peak time for rebleed is in the first 48 hours, with a second high-risk period occurring 7–10 days after the initial hemorrhage.

Systemic effects of subarachnoid hemorrhage are also quite common. Within hours of the initial hemorrhage, there is a release of catecholamines and cytokines. The catecholamine surge leads to increased heart rate and blood pressure and in some cases arrhythmias. Troponin levels rise for the first 6–8 hours after subarachnoid hemorrhage (Deibert et al., 2003; Hravnak et al., 2009), and arrhythmias are common in the first twelve hours including prolonged QT elevation, Q wave presence, ST elevation, and other arrhythmias (Wartenberg & Mayer, 2006). For most patients recovering from a subarachnoid hemorrhage, no long-term cardiac damage occurs and these signs and symptoms pass within the first 24 hours. Individuals with pre-hemorrhage cardiac disease or abnormalities may experience more severe cardiac consequences including heart attack and decreased ejection fraction. Cytokine release initiates an inflammatory response indicated by fever.

PREVENTION

There is limited literature on prevention of subarachnoid hemorrhage. Cerebral aneurysms are the most common cause of subarachnoid hemorrhage and are usually identifiable via Magnetic

Resonance Imaging (MRI). The cost of the MRI, coupled with the rarity of cerebral aneurysms, prohibits routine screening of patients. Current evidence suggests that screening should be performed on individuals with two or more first-degree relatives who have suffered aneurysmal subarachnoid hemorrhage. Individuals with autosomal dominant polycystic kidney disease who have had one first-degree relative with aneurysmal subarachnoid hemorrhage should be screened as well.

For individuals with a known cerebral aneurysm, basic lifestyle modifications may decrease risk. Certainly, anticoagulants and hypertension increase the risk of aneurysm rupture and subsequent subarachnoid hemorrhage. Cessation of cigarette smoking is of benefit as it is associated with higher risk for subarachnoid hemorrhage. Avoidance of cocaine or other substances known to increase blood pressure is also beneficial. A significant body of literature is developing to determine proper monitoring and ideal time for aneurysm securement. Small aneurysms – less than 5 mm – are less likely to rupture and may be managed through serial magnetic resonance imaging to monitor the size of aneurysm.

For individuals with a known AVM, serial MRI is warranted to monitor size and blood flow patterns through the AVM. AVM resection is generally warranted and usually is performed shortly after diagnosis to prevent hemorrhage and other effects/signs and symptoms due to blood diversion from healthy tissue into the AVM. Smoking cessation and blood pressure management are prudent measures for patients with known, unsecured AVMs.

Avoiding high-risk behaviors associated with head trauma is the only known way to decrease risk of subarachnoid hemorrhage due to trauma. Helmet use for bicycle and motorcycle riders, seat belts during vehicular transportation, and safe practices when climbing ladders or in other high areas should be recommended for all patients presenting to their health care professionals.

Uncontrolled hypertension, atherosclerosis, cocaine use, sickle cell disease (albeit more rarely), anticoagulant therapy, clotting disorders, and pituitary apoplexy have all been associated with subarachnoid hemorrhage. Maintaining good health habits with attention to cardiovascular health not only has heart health benefits but is likely to reduce risk of subarachnoid hemorrhage.

DIAGNOSIS

Diagnosis of subarachnoid hemorrhage begins with a clinical exam. Frequent symptoms include a sudden, severe headache, often termed a "thunderclap" headache due to the sudden increase in intracranial pressure. This type of headache is usually not relieved by over-the-counter pain medications such as aspirin or non-steroidal anti-inflammatory drugs. Brief loss of consciousness, nausea, and vomiting are common and caused by the sudden increase in intracranial pressure. Syncope is not an uncommon symptom of acute SAH. Blood in direct contact with the meninges leads to irritation and the symptoms of nuchal rigidity, lower back pain, and bilateral leg pain/discomfort. Visual anomalies such as photophobia and blurry or double vision are common due to cranial nerve irritation and damage. Motor deficits, often unilateral, due to middle cerebral artery involvement are noted in about 15% of patients. Seizures are fairly common, occurring in 10–20% of patients presenting with subarachnoid hemorrhage. Retinal hemorrhage and papilledema occur in a small percentage of patients due to increased intracranial pressure. Blood pressure is often elevated and/or labile due to catecholamine release and in response to elevated intracranial pressure.

In patients with suspected subarachnoid hemorrhage, prompt radiographic imaging to identify the source and extent of the bleeding is necessary. A cranial computed tomography (CT) scan with dye is the first test to be completed. Subarachnoid hemorrhage from different sources will exhibit different patterns. A circular or star-shaped hyperintensity near the center of the brain, the cisterns around the brainstem, and the basal cistern is diagnostic of ruptured cerebral aneurysm within one of the vessels of the Circle of Willis (see Figure 5.1). AVM rupture or leakage shows as a hyperintensity of the actual vessel abnormality and blood in the space nearby; however, AVMs can occur at various places within the brain. Traumatic subarachnoid hemorrhage often presents as widespread pockets of hyperintensity. A small subarachnoid hemorrhage or one greater than 8 days old may not be visible with a CT scan. For patients with an allergy to iodine, radiographic imaging should be undertaken with caution as dyes are iodine-based and may cause an acute allergic reaction. Allergic reactions to

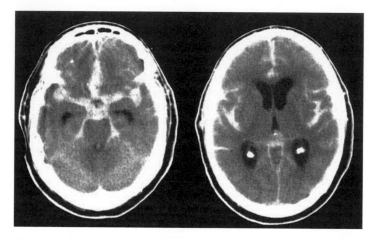

Fig. 5.1 CT scan showing aneurysmal subarachnoid hemorrhage. Reprinted with permission from Claassen J, Bernardini GL, Kreiter K, Bates J, Du YE, Copeland D, Connolly ES Jr, Mayer SA: Effect of cisternal ventricular blood on risk of delayed cerebral ischemia after subarachnoid hemorrhage: the Fisher scale revisited. Stroke 32:2012-2020, 2001, with permission from Lippincott Williams & Wilkins.

iodine-based dyes are often anaphylactic-type reactions leading to hives followed by cardiac and/or respiratory arrest.

If the CT scan does not show subarachnoid hemorrhage or is inconclusive, a lumbar puncture should be performed. Blood in the cerebrospinal fluid is indicative of subarachnoid hemorrhage. Typically, four tubes of CSF are drawn during a lumbar puncture. Blood in the first tube, and sometimes the second tube, generally appears due to the trauma of the procedure. Persistent blood in the third and fourth tubes indicates subarachnoid hemorrhage. Lumbar puncture is a painful procedure, with a risk of nerve damage and, in the case of lesions in the cranial area, herniation.

In patients with either a lumbar puncture indicative of subarachnoid hemorrhage or a CT scan indicative of subarachnoid hemorrhage without signs of obvious AVM, further testing is required to identify the source of hemorrhage. Computed tomography angiography (CTA) or cerebral angiography provides a more detailed visual description of the cerebral vasculature. These tests are used to identify location of AVMs and aneurysms. They provide the added benefit of showing position and shape of the abnormality that guide treatment options (see the subsection below on aneurysm securement).

If no vascular abnormality is found and the hemorrhage is not related to trauma, follow-up monitoring is still warranted and additional testing should occur to rule out aneurysm or AVM. Care and monitoring should occur as outlined below, although without further signs, symptoms, or positive test results, these patients may be transferred to a non-intensive care unit setting earlier and are typically discharged earlier. Additional MRI testing should be done 2–3 weeks after the hemorrhage, and again at 6 months and one year, to identify any additional vascular abnormalities.

ACUTE CARE

Once a diagnosis is confirmed, two common courses of action should occur. Often aneurysm or AVM coiling is performed in the angiogram suite immediately after diagnosis. For abnormalities not conducive to coil placement and securement, surgery is immediately performed for aneurysm or AVM securement. In other instances, vessel securement is postponed until the patient is more hemodynamically stable and proper staffing and equipment are available.

Aneurysm securement

The following section outlines pre-, intra-, and post-operative care of the patient having an aneurysm secured.

Pre-operative/pre-procedural care

If patients are not taken directly to the angiographic or surgical suite, they should be admitted to the intensive care unit. In the intensive care unit, care should be taken to minimize the risk of rebleed. The patient should be provided a quiet, dark environment to limit stimulation. Bed rest should be maintained and the patient should be encouraged not to strain/push to have a bowel movement or perform other behaviors that increase pressure in the cranial vault. There is no strong empirical evidence supporting a specific blood pressure range to prevent rebleed before aneurysm securement. Most clinicians agree systolic blood pressure should be maintained between 90 and 140 mmHg (Suarez, Tarr, & Selman, 2006). Analgesics often reduce blood pressure to an acceptable range. If analgesia is not effective in decreasing blood pressure within the target range, several vasoactive medications are acceptable. Labetalol, β-blockers, hydralazine, and nicardipine all have shown efficacy in safely controlling blood pressure within the target range after SAH (Diringer et al., 2011). Heart rate should be maintained within normal limits. Fever has been associated with poor outcome, so temperature should be maintained below 38.0°C with acetaminophen, ibuprofen, or surface cooling, if necessary. Acetaminophen and ibuprofen have limited efficacy in this population as fever is likely to result from a systemic inflammatory reaction, and a consensus report recommends continuous infusion of NSAIDS (diclofenac sodium) (Cormio & Citerio, 2007), newer surface cooling (Arctic Sun Temperature Management System, model 2000, Medivance, Louisville, CO) (Mayer et al., 2004), or intravascular cooling devices (Diringer et al., 2011). Oxygen should be administered as necessary to maintain PaO_2 at or above 90 mmHg. For patients who require intubation and mechanical ventilation, adequate sedation should be provided, suctioning should only be performed when needed, and positive-end-expiratory-pressure (PEEP) should be avoided as it decreases blood pressure and may result in cerebral ischemia (Muench et al., 2005).

Surgical management
Despite advancements in angiographic procedures, surgical clipping remains the most prominent form of aneurysm securement. During this surgical procedure, the surgeon must drill through the bone, remove a section of bone, and displace brain tissue to visualize the aneurysm. Once the aneurysm is visible, surgical clips are placed at the neck of the aneurysm to prevent blood from flowing into the aneurysm and the dome of the aneurysm is nicked to assure no blood enters the aneurysm. Historically, aneurysms were wrapped with gauze (to promote scar tissue formation around the aneurysm) or ligated for securement. While these procedures are rarely performed since the development of the surgical clip, there are times when they are preferable, providing a less dangerous procedure to the patient or more effective securement of the aneurysm. Aneurysms in the anterior circulation and berry-type aneurysms

are more amenable to surgical clipping. Patients having surgical securement of cerebral aneurysms are still at risk for complications commonly associated with anesthesia and surgery, including infection.

Post-operative care

Patients recovering from brain surgery for aneurysm securement require an intensive care unit setting. Once the aneurysm has been secured, certain limitations may be released. A target blood pressure of less than 200 mmHg is ideal to allow adequate cerebral perfusion once the risk of aneurysm rupture has been removed (Suarez, Tarr, & Selman, 2006), although this is based on expert opinion rather than empirical evidence. Ventilator management can include more frequent suctioning, although PEEP should still be avoided. Frequent neurologic assessment should be performed (every 1-2 hours) to monitor for complications, potential rebleed, cerebral edema, and untoward anesthesia effects.

Coil embolization

Some patients may not be hemodynamically stable enough for surgery. Some aneurysms are not amenable to surgical clipping due to location, position, or shape. Recent evidence has shown that coil embolization of aneurysms in patients in good pre-rupture health is associated with higher survival rates and increased independence (Van der Schaaf et al., 2009). Whether this relates to decreased risk infection, reduction of anesthesia required for embolization, or some other factor is unclear. Fusiform aneurysms and berry aneurysms (see Figure 5.2) with a wide neck are difficult to treat with a surgical clip. Aneurysms within the posterior circulation are more difficult to treat surgically as more brain must be displaced to reach the aneurysm. In circumstances where surgery is not likely to be safe or effective in securing the aneurysm, coil embolization is often a safe and effective alternative. The development of coil embolization in 1991 has significantly improved outcome for patients who are high surgical risks or have aneurysms that cannot be secured with typical surgical techniques. While this is a relatively new procedure, evidence supports it is as safe and effective for aneurysm securement, and it is associated with similar outcomes to patients undergoing surgical aneurysm securement.

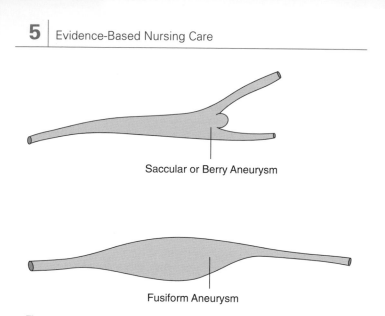

Saccular or Berry Aneurysm

Fusiform Aneurysm

Fig. 5.2 Structures of the most common aneurysm types.

Coil embolization is performed by a neurosurgeon or an interventional neuroradiologist who has had additional training in this procedure. An angiographic catheter is threaded through the femoral artery into the internal carotid artery and up into the cranial vault during typical angiography. Radio-opaque dye is injected into the vessels and fills distal vessels, thereby identifying vascular abnormalities that fill with dye. Once the location and position of the aneurysm has been identified, the decision is made to take the patient to surgery for clipping of the aneurysm or coil embolization in the angiogram suite. For patients undergoing coil embolization, a catheter is threaded through the vessels and into the aneurysm. A charge of electricity travels through the catheter and releases the coil into the aneurysm. This procedure must be performed repeatedly until the aneurysm is filled with coils. Finally, an additional electric charge is transmitted through the catheter to initiate blood coagulation. Once the aneurysm is filled with coils, blood no longer flows through the aneurysm and it is no longer at risk of rupture. Coil embolization assumes the same risks as traditional cerebral angiography, including hemorrhage due to puncture of a vessel, hematoma formation at the catheterization site, anesthesia-related complications and infection, or release of coils outside the aneurysm, although less anesthesia is used and infection risk is lower as compared to surgical management.

Post-procedural care

Patients recovering from coil embolization require care in an intensive care unit setting. Once the aneurysm has been secured, certain limitations may be released. A target blood pressure of less than 200 mmHg is ideal to allow adequate cerebral perfusion once the risk of aneurysm rupture has been removed. Ventilator management can include more frequent suctioning, although PEEP should still be avoided. Frequent neurologic assessment should be performed (every 1–2 hours) to monitor for complications, potential rebleed, cerebral edema, and untoward anesthesia effects. If the angiographic catheter has been left in the patient, it should be connected to a pressure monitor with alarm settings set to identify blood pressure greater than the upper limit identified above, but also to identify a significant drop in blood pressure that could impair cerebral perfusion and catheter disconnect/dislodgement. Angiographic catheters are large and can lead to significant bleeding if dislodged. A properly placed catheter can leak and lead to hematoma formation. Catheter placement site should be covered with an occlusive dressing, and the insertion site should be monitored periodically (every 5–15 minutes for the first 1–2 hours, then every 1–2 hours until removal) for leakage or hematoma. If blood is to be drawn from this line, sterile blood draw procedures should be used and care should be taken to prevent catheter dislodgement.

Other management approaches

For a small number of patients with subarachnoid hemorrhage due to an aneurysm rupture, neither surgical nor coil embolization is possible. In these patients, monitoring is vital to identify change as quickly as possible and prevent damage.

AVM securement

There is minimal evidence identifying the ideal management of an unruptured AVM. The risk of AVM is fairly low at about 1–4%

with significant variance by population reported. Clinical sequelae from AVMs are often mild, not causing the patient to seek care. The rupture of an AVM leading to intraparenchymal hemorrhage, SAH, or intraventricular hemorrhage is seen as the initial, presenting symptom in more than 50% of AVMs (Fults & Kelly, 1984). Most commonly, ruptured AVMs result in intraparenchymal hemorrhage. For patients with SAH from ruptured AVM, the risk of severe cerebral vasospasm is extremely low.

There is evidence supporting medical management, surgical management, and interventional radiologic methods to treat AVMs, but there is no empirical evidence showing superior efficacy of any method. There is evidence showing that surgical and radiologic interventional methods carry a risk of intraparenchymal and subarachnoid hemorrhage. Patients having AVM securement via surgical resection, embolization, or radiosurgery should be monitored closely for subarachnoid and intraparenchymal hemorrhage. There is risk of a hemorrhagic event during or due to interventional treatment, which may be greater than risk of rupture of an AVM without treatment. Risk of other stroke or injury during or after treatment is not insignificant, and those receiving treatment have a higher risk of disability. This data is difficult to interpret given that there are not clear guidelines at this time as to which AVMs are likely to rupture leading to devastating consequences versus mild consequences. Anatomical location, size of AVM, vessel integrity, co-morbid conditions, and patient age all contribute to risk of AVM rupture, potential disability from rupture, and treatment options available. While there is decreased risk of cerebral vasospasm from ruptured AVMs due to treatment, the risk of most other side effects remains the same. Once an AVM has ruptured, some form of treatment is definitely warranted. The risk of rebleed from a previously ruptured AVM without treatment/securement/ablation is significant (up to 25%). Once an AVM has been resected, outcome is directly correlated with size, location, and deep venous drainage, with larger, more complex AVMs having a higher risk of poor outcomes.

Pre-treatment and post-treatment care guidelines provided below are focused on AVM's that have ruptured without treatment, however they can and should be applied to patients suffering ruptured AVM during securement procedures.

AVM resection
Preoperative/pre-procedural care
In many instances, a patient with a ruptured AVM will be taken directly to the operating room or radiology suite for treatment. Typically, the clot is removed, and if the AVM is superficial it may be resected. If the AVM is deep and/or complicated, the clot is typically removed and the AVM is left intact for future stabilization. Many surgeons prefer to remove only the clot and leave the AVM intact for future removal. If patients are not taken directly to the angiographic or surgical suite they should be admitted to the intensive care unit. In the intensive care unit, care should be taken to minimize the risk of rebleed. The patient should be provided a quiet, dark environment to limit stimulation. Bed rest should be maintained and the patient should be encouraged not to strain/push to have a bowel movement or perform other behaviors that increase pressure in the cranial vault. Blood pressure and heart rate should generally be maintained at a normal level for the patient. Temperature should be maintained below $38.0°C$ with acetaminophen, ibuprofen, or surface cooling if necessary. Oxygen should be administered as necessary to maintain PaO_2 above 90. For patients who require intubation and mechanical ventilation, adequate sedation should be provided.

Surgical management
Surgical resection is the most common treatment modality used to treat ruptured AVMs. It is an operative procedure involving the removal of a portion of the skull and the displacement of brain tissue until the AVM is visualized. The arterial feeders to the AVM are resected first, followed by the nidus (central portion of the AVM) and then the venous drainage vessel(s). Advancements in surgical care have decreased surgical side effects due to displacement of brain tissue, as microsurgical techniques permit less displacement of tissue. The goal of surgical resection of the AVM is complete obliteration, but if this is not possible, other techniques may be employed. Intra- or postoperative angiography should be utilized to verify complete obliteration to prevent subsequent hemorrhage. For AVMs that are not completely obliterated during the surgical procedure, there is risk of rebleed until the AVM is obliterated.

In the operative period, anesthetics and vasoactive agents that cause cerebral vasodilation should be avoided. Euvolemia, normotension, isotension, normoglycemia, and mild hypocapnia are recommended. Normothermia is currently recommended although ongoing studies are exploring the efficacy of hypothermia during intracranial surgeries including AVM obliteration. Hypotension should be considered for surgical treatment of AVMs with a deep arterial supply. Intra-operative and acute post-operative hemorrhage or edema may be due to a hyperemic state. In cases where hyperemia is present and severe, α-adrenergic blockade may be utilized.

Postoperative care

Initial postoperative care of the patient having surgical resection of an AVM includes frequent vital sign monitoring and neurologic assessment. Postoperative AVM resection patients should be admitted to a neurological/neurosurgical intensive care unit for a minimum of 24 hours after surgery. Rebleed of the AVM in the first week after surgical resection occurs in about 10% of patients. Risk of rebleed in the first year has been estimated at 6–18%, and then decreases to 3–4%. In the postoperative period, acute changes in neurologic examination remain the most common and effective way to identify rebleed. Hemodynamic stability is of vital importance after surgical resection of an AVM. If intracranial pressure is being monitored, it should be maintained below 20 mmHg. As with most neurosurgical patients, cerebral perfusion pressure should be maintained above 60 mmHg to ensure adequate oxygen and nutrient delivery. If CPP is above 60 mmHg, frequent neurologic assessment is still required. Regional decreases in blood flow delivery can lead to less than optimal delivery to areas near the AVM, and hypoxia, ischemia, and neuronal cell death can occur. Any new neurologic deficit warrants a CT scan to rule out hemorrhage or hydrocephalus. Blood pressure should be maintained at the patient's normal pressure. If needed, mean arterial pressure MAP should be treated with medications that do not act on the central nervous system. Urine output should be tightly monitored and euvolemia should be maintained.

Endovascular treatment

Particularly large and/or complex AVMs may not be amenable to surgical treatment alone. Endovascular treatment of an AVM includes embolization and/or coiling of aneurysms in vessels feeding the AVM. Embolization involves administration of polyvinyl alcohol particles, fibers, microcoils, microballoons, cyanoacrylate monomers, polymer solutions, and absolute ethanol. AVM size is often reduced in this manner before surgical or radiosurgical treatment is performed to completely obliterate the AVM. In some instances, endovascular treatment is used to obliterate AVM remnants after partial surgical obliteration. In select patients with large, inoperable cortical and subcortical AVMs and in patients presenting with seizures resistant to medical management or with progressive neurological deficit thought to be secondary to venous hypertension and/or arterial steal, endovascular treatment may be employed to decrease signs and symptoms. In these instances embolization usually only partly obliterates the AVM and relief of signs and symptoms is often temporary. In particularly small, simple AVMs endovascular treatment may be used as the only therapeutic modality. In patients where this is the only therapy applied to AVM obliteration, follow up should include periodic angiograms to monitor for recanalization of the AVM.

Both general anesthesia and deep intravenous sedation are currently used during endovascular procedures for AVM treatment. Currently there is no empirical evidence showing improved efficacy of either method. Deep intravenous sedation permits the opportunity to intermittently examine select neurologic function as necessary. During the endovascular procedure, a large intra-arterial catheter will be placed in the femoral artery for monitoring of blood pressure. Hypotension may be induced with vasoactive agents, general anesthetics, or brief adenosine-induced cardiac pause during select periods of the procedure. Hypotension permits more accurate deposition of substances into the nidus of the AVM. A pulse oximeter should be placed to monitor systemic oxygenation, with a second pulse oximeter placed on the extremity distal to the arterial puncture site. The extremity distal to the puncture site is at increased risk for femoral artery obstruction and distal thromboembolism. Coagulation status of the patient should be considered.

Anticoagulation with heparin is frequently used to prevent thromboembolic complications.

Post-procedural care

Frequent neurologic assessment is required after endovascular treatment of an AVM. While the AVM is generally secure if fully embolized, there is the possibility of displacement of embolization materials into other vessels, leading to alterations (decreases) in blood flow and potential stroke to new areas of brain. In the very-early-phase post-treatment, an acute change in level of consciousness may indicate there has been mechanical injury to the cerebral vessels resulting in rebleed. Pulse oximeter monitoring of the extremity distal to the puncture site should continue to persistant risk of femoral artery obstruction, distal thromboembolism and the additional risk of ischemia due to overcompression in the acute post-procedural period. Urinary catheters are recommended for monitoring output and patient comfort and to decrease the risk of hematoma. Supplemental oxygen and/or ventilator support should be considered in the context of the patient's general health and sedative administration. The need for anticoagulation to prevent thromboembolic complications should be considered. While there is currently no consistent recommendation for a specific algorithm for anticoagulation of patients post-AVM treatment, it is generally recommended that these patients should be anticoagulated with heparin before the procedure and for the acute post-procedure period.

Other management approaches
Radiotherapy

Radiotherapy involves administering focal doses of radiation in an effort to reduce or fully ablate the abnormal vessel. Typically, radiotherapy is used for small, unruptured AVMs because it requires repeat doses/treatments to achieve any decreased flow in the AVM and decrease risk of rebleed.

Support of hemodynamic stability
Neurologic

Frequent and often invasive monitoring is needed to identify problems early and maximize outcome after subarachnoid hemorrhage. Neurologic examination identifies dysfunction of brain tissue and often serves as the only warning of impending stroke. Signs/symptoms identified early after their onset permit medical and/or surgical intervention to treat the underlying problem and limit tissue damage or death, thereby maximizing functional recovery. Any change in neurologic examination warrants notification of additional health care providers including the nurse practitioner, resident, and/or attending physician depending on the infrastructure and policies in the setting where care is being provided. A full neurologic examination should be performed on all patients upon admission to the post-anesthesia care unit (if used) and intensive care unit, and then every hour for the first 8 hours after admission.

Patients with known, unsecured aneurysms or AVMs should have full neurologic examination performed every 8 hours, with a brief focused examination occurring every hour until the aneurysm is secured. This focused neurologic examination should include an assessment of level of consciousness, orientation, visual field assessment, cranial nerve assessment except for testing cough and gag reflexes (cranial nerves IX and X) due to risk of increased intracranial pressure and rupture, and motor strength/sensation of all four extremities. If surgery is delayed for a significant period of time – more than two days – neurologic examinations must be balanced with the patients' need for rest and sleep and may be decreased to every 2 to 4 hours.

For patients with secured aneurysms, frequency of neurologic assessments may be tailored based on risk. During the early postoperative/post-procedural period, a complete neurologic examination should occur every hour for the first 8 to 12 hours after surgery. For patients who have awakened from anesthesia and are responsive 8–12 hours after surgery/procedure, complete neurologic assessment may be decreased to every 2 hours until 96 hours after hemorrhage. If that patient is still stable and without signs of complications 96 hours after hemorrhage, complete neurologic assessments should be performed every 4 hours through 7 to 10 days after hemorrhage.

Managing and monitoring intracranial pressure

Many catheters are available to monitor tissue-level changes in intracranial pressure, and brain perfusion, temperature, oxygen, and other substrate release indicative of pending tissue damage. Intracranial pressure is the force applied to brain tissue by the contents of the skull. The skull is not pliable and only able to hold a certain volume. When there is an increase in blood, cerebrospinal fluid, or brain tissue, the other two substances must decrease to accommodate the increase in volume in the skull. Neurologic examination identifies increases in intracranial pressure (see Table 5.1 for signs/symptoms of increased intracranial pressure) but generally identifies tissue being damaged and at risk for death. Invasive monitoring permits identification of small increases in intracranial pressure before tissue death occurs. Intracranial pressure monitoring is performed with one of three different monitors.

Subdural and subarachnoid screws/bolts

This device consists of a hollow bolt or screw that is inserted through a hole made in the bone and dura. The end of the bolt (or screw) lays against the arachnoid and senses intracranial pressure. These devices permit monitoring of intracranial pressure but do not permit drainage of fluid. The risk associated with screws/bolts is primarily related to infection, because the dura has been breached and bacteria can more easily gain access to the central nervous system.

Intraventricular catheters

These catheters are inserted through a hole in the skull and dura, tunneled through the brain tissue into the lateral ventricles. They measure the pressure inside the ventricles and are the most accurate pressure monitors. Intraventricular catheters are an attractive tool as they permit drainage of cerebrospinal fluid out of the ventricles through the catheter to facilitate intracranial pressure management. They carry significant risk of potential brain damage during placement and infection, because barriers between central nervous system and external environment are breached.

Intraparenchymal catheters

Intraparenchymal catheters are inserted through a hole in the skull, dura, arachnoid, and pia. The catheter is inserted into the brain tissue. These catheters are often coupled with blood flow monitors providing additional monitoring information. These catheters provide a more accurate measure of intracranial pressure but do not

Table 5.1 Signs and symptoms of increased intracranial pressure

	Sign/symptom	Level of damage
Early findings (mild increase in ICP)	Headache	Cortex
	Altered level of consciousness – drowsiness, restlessness, lethargy	Cortex/global pressure
	Decreased visual acuity	Cranial nerve II
	Blurry vision	
	Papilledema	Cranial nerve II
	Small pupils to early dilation AND/OR	Cranial nerve III
	Ovoid with a sluggish response AND/OR	
	Hippus response to light	
	These papillary changes are often present on side ipsilateral to the edema/ lesion.	
	Motor weakness (monoparesis or hemiparesis)	Motor cortex and pyramidal tract
Mid-level findings (moderate increase in ICP)	Increased blood pressure	Cortex/compensatory mechanism
	Progressive decrease in level of consciousness	Cortex/global pressure
	More pronounced visual acuity/clarity deficits	Cranial nerve II
	Impaired pupil response to light	Midbrain
	Disconjugate gaze (CN)	Pons
	Projectile vomiting	Area postrema (vomiting center) in the Medulla
	Cushing's response (increased systolic blood pressure, widened pulse pressure, decreased heart rate)	Compensatory mechanism
Late findings (Severe increase in ICP)	Further decrease in level of consciousness to unresponsive to stimulation	Cortex/global pressure
	Loss of brain stem reflexes	Brainstem
	Decorticate and decerebrate posturing	Brainstem
	Weak, irregular, rapid heart rate, respiratory rate	Global

provide a mechanism for fluid removal or treatment. While there is risk of brain damage during placement, the catheter is very small and resides in a superficial area of the brain, so minimal damage is to be expected with proper placement. Infection risk remains significant as the barriers between central nervous system and external environment are breached.

Secondary injury

Secondary injury from rebleed, cerebral vasospasm, hydrocephalus, and cerebral edema is a common occurrence after subarachnoid hemorrhage. Neurologic monitoring can detect a pending insult and permit adequate time to initiate treatment and limit damage/deficit. Various monitoring devices in combination with frequent neurologic and vital sign assessment aid the nurse in the critical care arena in maximizing outcome for patients.

Rebleeding

Monitoring for aneurysm rebleed is vital in patients with an unsecured aneurysm. In patients who have multiple aneurysms, of which not all have been secured, frequent neurologic exam and monitoring may identify additional bleeding. While it is vital to support CPP during the acute period, this often must be balanced with maintaining a blood pressure that will inhibit rupture of any aneurysm, leakage of blood from an AVM, or rebleeding of unsecured aneurysms or AVMs. Coughing, straining, and sharp elevations in blood pressure should be avoided.

Cerebral vasospasm and delayed cerebral ischemia

Cerebral vasospasm, a spasm of one or more cerebral vessels decreasing the internal lumen of the vessel, is one of the most common complications of aneurysmal subarachnoid hemorrhage. Delayed cerebral ischemia (DCI) occurs when ischemia develops days after aneurysmal subarachnoid hemorrhage, often in association with cerebral vasospasm. While significantly less common in patients recovering from subarachnoid hemorrhage due to other sources, the majority of subarachnoid hemorrhages is due to a ruptured cerebral aneurysm, and they are at risk for cerebral vasospasm and DCI. Spasm of a cerebral blood vessel leads to a decrease in internal lumen size and blood delivery to brain tissue. Symptoms of cerebral vasospasm and DCI range from non-existent to severe deficit and are directly related to the brain tissue suffering hypoxia and/or ischemia. Treatment of cerebral vasospasm and DCI is focused on maintaining adequate cerebral perfusion pressure through local and systemic vascular support.

Calcium channel blockers

Calcium channel blockers or antagonists have shown some success in preventing long-term deficits from cerebral vasospasm and DCI. Nimodipine is the most commonly used calcium channel blocker to prevent cerebral vasospasm and improve outcomes from aneurysmal SAH. Nimodipine and other calcium channel blockers are thought to prevent calcium entry into the smooth muscle cells of the blood vessels, thereby preventing constriction. Nimodipine has shown primary actions on the cerebral vasculature with limited systemic activity. Despite this hypothesized mechanism of action, clinical trials of nimodipine after aneurysmal subarachnoid hemorrhage did not show significant reduction in angiographic vessel size. Additional research has suggested that nimodipine administration decreases the severity of neurologic deficits after subarachnoid hemorrhage. Nimodipine should be administered at a dose of 60 mg orally or via nasogastric tube every 4 hours for the first 21 days after subarachnoid hemorrhage. It should be given at least 1 hour before and 2 hours after meals. Nimodipine should *not* be administered intravenously or via other parenteral routes as this can result in severe drop in blood pressure, bradycardia, cardiovascular collapse, cardiac arrest, and death. Side effects of nimodipine are rare but include a drop in systolic blood pressure. Patients experiencing an unsafe drop in blood pressure after taking a full dose of nimodipine may better tolerate dosing of 30 mg orally or via nasogastric tube every 2 to 4 hours for 21 days. Nimodipine metabolism is decreased in patients with impaired hepatic function. Patients with impaired hepatic function should be trialed on a lower dose of nimodipine, and heart rate and blood pressure should be monitored more closely for instability.

Other calcium channel blockers may be used to maintain adequate blood pressure and cerebral perfusion pressure; however, they should be added to Nimodipine therapy. The questionable mechanism of action and the association with improved long-term outcomes support the use of Nimodipine as an independent treatment to improve functional recovery after aneurysmal subarachnoid hemorrhage.

Endothelin receptor antagonists

Bosentan is a dual endothelin receptor antagonist targeting both endothelin-A and endothelin-B receptors. Bosentan induces arterial relaxation by blocking the effects of endothelin at the level of the cerebral vasculature. High-dose Bosentan (up to 40 mg/kg/day) for up to 14 days has been shown to be safe for patients recovering from SAH (Clozel, 2000; Nogueira et al., 2007). While safety has been established, efficacy of this drug to prevent cerebral vasospasm and DCI after SAH is under investigation and no definitive recommendation can be made at this time. Use of Bosentan in patients with impaired liver function should be carefully considered due to potential hepatotoxicity. Liver function tests should be monitored. It is contraindicated in pregnant women due to teratogenic effects.

Clazosentan is an endothelin receptor antagonist. It was developed to target the endothelin-A receptor and optimize aqueous solubility. Doses of 5–15 mg/hour have been proposed to decrease incidence of cerebral vasospasm in aneurysmal SAH patients. A phase III trial of clazosentan effects on cerebral vasospasm and outcome from SAH did not show efficacy (Macdonald et al., 2011).

Magnesium

Magnesium (Mg) is a non-competitive voltage-dependent calcium channel antagonist. It also inhibits excitatory amino acid release and blocks N-methyl D-aspartate receptors. Mg induces cerebral vasodilation (Pyne, Cadoux-Hudson, & Clark, 2001). In a rat model, Mg administration reduced cerebral vasospasm and infarct size (Ram et al., 1991; Marinov et al., 1996; van den Berg, 2002). Recent evidence suggests that magnesium supplementation may decrease incidence and severity of cerebral vasospasm in humans as well. A 2005 randomized clinical trial (RCT) by van Norden, van den Bergh, and Rinkel (2005) found that subjects randomized to receive 64 mMol Mg per day had a 34% DCI risk reduction. The decrease in cerebral vasospasm/DCI and improved outcomes in aSAH patients has been shown in other studies (Veyna et al., 2002; Muroi et al., 2008). Dose-response studies have shown that 64 mMol of Mg/day maintained serum Mg within the 1.0–2.0 mMol/L range (van den Berg et al., 2003; van Norden et al., 2005). Follow-up work in a meta-analysis concluded that IV Mg reduced risk of DCI (relative risk 0.73, 95% CI 0.53–1.00) and poor outcome (relative risk 0.62, 95% CI 0.46–0.83) (Ma et al., 2010).

While this evidence shows Mg therapy is a safe and effective treatment to minimize neurologic damage and improve outcome after aSAH, there are some side effects that should be monitored. The overall goal of Mg therapy should be to maintain serum Mg levels between 1.0 and 2.0 mg/L and daily Mg levels should be monitored. Daily calcium should also be monitored, as Mg supplementation has been shown to increase risk of hypocalcemia (Veyna et al., 2002; Muroi et al., 2008), although this hypocalcemia has not been associated with neuromuscular irritability, DCI/vasospasm, or poor outcomes (Veyna et al., 2002; Muroi et al., 2008; van den Bergh et al., 2008). Mg intoxication can occur with levels above 2.5 mMol/L, producing such symptoms as nausea, headache, flushed feeling, drowsiness, hypotension, hypocalcemia, hyperkalemia, respiratory arrest, and cardiac arrhythmias including PR and QRS prolongation, cardiac depression, AV block, and cardiac arrest. Patients receiving Mg therapy should be monitored for hypotension and arrhythmias (Ma et al., 2010). Finally, renal function should be monitored as renal failure has been associated with continuous Mg infusion and elevated Mg levels (van Norden et al., 2005).

Triple H therapy

Triple H therapy (HHH) incorporates hypervolemia, hypertension, and hemodilution to increase cerebral blood flow and circulation, increase cardiac output, maximize cerebral perfusion pressure, and ultimately decrease ischemic deficits related to cerebral vasospasm. Goals of HHH are to maintain CVP at 8–12 mmHg, hematocrit below 30, and systolic blood pressure between 160 and 200 mmHg (Kassell et al., 1982; Muizelaar & Becker, 1986; Awad et al., 1987). Hemodilution (hematocrit below 30) has been shown not to be effective and it may be detrimental to patient outcomes, so it is not recommended for routine use in this population. Crystalloid or colloid infusion and pharmacologic agents are thought to be equally effective in achieving these goals (Janjua & Mayer, 2003). While HHH therapy may be instituted as a prophylactic therapy in aSAH patients, it is more often used in response to suspected or diagnosed cerebral vasospasm and DCI. Individual components of this therapy may also be used to maximize cerebral blood flow and perfusion. Patients with elevated transcranial Doppler ultrasonography values, suggesting cerebral vasospasm, or other evidence of cerebral vasospasm but without clinical signs/symptoms should have, at a minimum, CVP monitoring with crystalloid fluid bolus to maintain it at or above 8 mmHg. Caution should be taken in patients with underlying cardiac disease, as the increase in fluid volume can exacerbate conditions such as heart failure. In patients with severe cardiac co-morbidities, pulmonary artery wedge pressure and cardiac index may be used to guide therapy. Specifically, fluid should be administered to maintain pulmonary artery wedge pressure above 12 mmHg and cardiac index above 4 L/min.

Intra-arterial therapies
When HHH therapy is not effective at decreasing cerebral vasospasm or DCI, additional therapies are warranted. Intra-arterial injectable therapies offer an additional tool to provide local dilation of the cerebral vessels. A cerebral angiogram is utilized to identify spastic cerebral vessels, and a vasodilatory drug is injected at the site of the vasospasm, or the vessel is manually opened with balloon angioplasty. Papavarine is an agent that has been used favorably to reduce local cerebral vasospasm. Other agents have been shown to be effective as well (Table 5.2).

Care of the patient post-cerebral angiogram for either transluminal balloon angioplasty or intra-arterial medication administration is similar to that for the care of any post-angiography patient. Frequent monitoring (every 1–2 hours) of the catheter placement site, vital signs, and neurologic examination is warranted. The bedside nurse should monitor the catheter placement site for signs of hematoma or active bleeding. Vital signs should be monitored for signs of blood loss and hemodynamic instability after the administration of intra-arterial medications. Neurologic examination is warranted to monitor for improvement in exam related to the treatment and decline in exam related to vessel perforation during the procedure, adverse reaction to the administered medication, and further vasospasm.

Table 5.2 Intra-arterial agents used fro the treatment of cerebral vasospasm

Agent	Class/Level of evidence	Mechanism of action	Usage/limitations	References
Papaverine	Class II/ Level 2	Opium alkaloid	Ventricular arrhythmia as a side effect.	Fandino, J., Kaku, Y., Schuknecht, B., Valavanis, A., & Yonekawa, Y. (1998). Improvement of cerebral oxygenation patterns and metabolic validation of superselective intra-arterial infusion of papaverine for the treatment of cerebral vasospasm. *Journal of Neurosurgery, 89*(1), 93–100. Kaku, Y., Yonekawa, Y., Tsukahara, T., & Kazekawa, K. (1992). Superselective intra-arterial infusion of papaverine for the treatment of cerebral vasospasm after subarachnoid hemorrhage. *Journal of Neurosurgery, 77*(6), 842–847. Polin, R. S., Hansen, C. A., German, P., Chadduck, J. P., & Kassell, N. F. (1998). Intra-arterially administered papaverine for the treatment of symptomatic cerebral vasospasm. *Neurosurgery, 42*(6), 1256–1264. Sawada, M., Hashimoto, N., Tsukahara, T., Nishi, S., Kaku, Y., & Yoshimura, S. (1997). Effectiveness of intra-arterial infused papavarine solutions of various concentrations for the treatment of cerebral vasospasm. *Acta Neurochirurgica, 139*(8), 706–711.

(Continued)

Table 5.2 (*Continued*)

Agent	Class/Level of evidence	Mechanism of action	Usage/limitations	References
				Clouston, J. E., Numaguchi, Y., Zoarski, G. H., Aldrich, E. F., Simard, J. M., & Zitnay, K. M. (1995). Intra-arterial papaverine infusion for cerebral vasospasm after subarachnoid hemorrhage. *American Journal of Neuroradiology, 16*, 27–38.
Verapamil	Class II/ Level 2	Calcium channel blocker, L-type		Sehy, J. V., Holloway, W. E., Lin, S.-P., Cross III, D. T., Derdeyn, C. P., & Moran, C. J. (2010). Improvement in angiographic cerebral vasospasm after intra-arterial verapamil administration. *American Journal of Neuroradiology, 31*, 1923–1928.
Nicardipine (Cardene)	Class II/ Level 2	Calcium channel blocker, L-type	Dose response hypotension	Rosenberg, N., Lazzaro, M. A., Lopes, D. K., & Prabhakaran, S. (2011). High-dose intra-arterial nicardipine results in hypotension following vasospasm treatment in aSAH. *Neurocritical Care, 15*(3), 400–404.
				Nogueira, R. G., Lev, M. H., Roccatagliata, L., Hirsch, J. A., Gonzalez, R. J., Ogilvy, C. S., Halpern, E. F., Rordorf, G. A., Rabinov, J. D., & J.C. Pryor. (2009). Intra-arterial nicardipine infusion improves CT perfusion-measured cerebral blood flow in patients with subarachnoid hemorrhage-induced vasospasm. *American Journal of Neuroradiology, 30*, 160–164.

Nimodipine (Nimotop)	Class II/ Level 2	Calcium channel blocker, L-type	Efficacy greater than papavarine in severe, refractory cerebral vasospasm. Short acting.	Hanggi, D., Turowski, B., Beseoglu, K., Yong, M., & Steiger, H. F. (2008). Intra-arterial nimodipine for severe cerebral vasospasm after aSAH: Influence on clinical course and cerebral perfusion. *American Journal of Neuroradiology, 29,* 1053–1060.
				Kurtz, P. M. P., Falcao, C. H. E., Magalhaes, M. D., Terrana, D., Prado, D. A., & Souza, P. C. P. (2005). Effect of intra-arterial nimodipine in patients with subarachnoid hemorrhage and refractory vasospasm: A pilot study. *Critical Care, 9*(S2), 94.
				Biondi, A., Ricciardi, G. K., Puybasset, L., Abdennour, L., Longo, M., Chiras, J., & Van Effenterre, R. (2004). Intra-arterial nimodipine for the treatment of symptomatic cerebral vasospasm after aneurysmal subarachnoid hemorrhage: Preliminary results. *American Journal of Neuroradiology, 25,* 1067–1076.
Fasudil Hydrochloride	Class II/ Level 2 Class I/ Level 1	Rho-kinase inhibitor Vasodilator		Tanaka, K., Minami, H., Kota, M., Kuwamura, K., & Kohmura, E. (2005). Treatment of cerebral vasospasm with intra-arterial fasudil hydrochloride. *Neurosurgery, 56*(2), 214–223.
				Tachibana, E., Harada, T., Shibuya, M., Saito, K., Takayasu, M., Suzuki, Y., et al. (1999). Intra-arterial infusion of fasudil hydrochloride for treating vasospasm following subarachnoid haemorrhage. *Acta Neurochirurgica, 141*(1), 13–19.

(Continued)

Table 5.2 (*Continued*)

Agent	Class/Level of evidence	Mechanism of action	Usage/limitations	References
				Shibuya, M., Suzuki, Y., Sugita, K., Saito, I., Sasaki, T., Takakura, K., et al. (1992). Effect of AT877 on cerebral vasospasm after aneurysmal subarachnoid hemorrhage: Results of a prospective placebo-controlled double-blind trial. *Journal of Neurosurgery, 76,* 571–577.
Milrinone (Primacore)	Class II/ Level 2	Phospho-diesterase inhibitor	Minimal research, although it appears efficacious. Possible side effects include ventricular arrhythmias.	Shankar, J. J., dos Santos, M. P., Deus-Silva, L., & Lum, C. (2011). Angiographic evaluation of the effect of intra-arterial milrinone therapy in patients with vasospasm from aneurysmal subarachnoid hemorrhage. *Neuroradiology, 53*(2), 123–128.
Nicardipine and papavarine	Class II/ Level 2	See above.	Efficacious, although not superior to papavarine alone.	Yoshimura, S., Tsukahara, T., Hashimoto, N., Kazekawa, K., & Kobayashi, A. (1995). Intra-arterial infusion of papaverine combined with intravenous administration of high-dose nicardipine for cerebral vasospasm. *Acta Neurochirurgica, 135*(3–4), 186–190.
Mg in combination with nicardipine	Class II/ Level 2	See above.		Shah, Q. A., Memon, M. Z., Fareed, M., Sari, K., Rodriguez, G. J., Kozak, O., Taylor, R. A., Tummala, R. P., Vazquez, G., Georgiadis, A. L., & Quereshi, A. I. (2009). Super-selective intra-arterial magnesium sulfate in combination with nicardipine for treatment of cerebral vasospasm in patients with subarachnoid hemorrhage. *Neurocritical Care, 11,* 190–198.

Hydrocephalus

Hydrocephalus is an enlargement of the cerebral ventricles due to increased volume of cerebrospinal fluid. It is a common complication of SAH and occurs in about 30% of patients. It presents as an abrupt decrease in level of consciousness with increasing neurologic dysfunction resulting in coma and ultimately death if untreated. Intracranial pressure due to hydrocephalus is often managed via ventriculostomy in the acute phase. For refractory increases in ICP, mannitol and, in some severe circumstances, hypertonic saline can decrease pressure and alleviate the pathology driving the symptoms of hydrocephalus.

Hydrocephalus occurs later in the recovery period, more than 10 days after admission, from SAH as well. In up to 15% of patients, a chronic hydrocephalus will develop due to blockage of the ventricular drainage system by blood (Demirgil et al., 2003). Obstruction of the ventricular system traps cerebrospinal fluid within the lateral and third ventricles, where it is produced. In rare instances, and often in the case of traumatic SAH, blood clots along the superior sagittal sinus, obstructing cerebrospinal fluid absorption. The result is an increase in fluid within the cranial vault and pressure on the brain. This more chronic form of hydrocephalus presents as unstable gait, incontinence, and altered cognitive functioning. Treatment of chronic hydrocephalus requires shunt placement to displace cerebrospinal fluid. A shunt is placed connecting the lateral ventricles and the abdomen. Most shunts have a valve blocking retrograde flow. When excess cerebrospinal fluid exerts pressure on the brain, causing an increase in intracranial pressure, the fluid will enter the shunt and drain into the abdominal cavity where it is absorbed.

Hyponatremia

Hyponatremia, due to renal loss during cerebral salt wasting, occurs in up to 30% of aneurysmal SAH patients and leads to worse outcome (Doczi et al., 1981; Qureshi et al., 2002). The hypo-osmolar state resulting from this serum hyponatremia alters blood brain barrier dynamics and results in cerebral edema. The hypo-osmolar state also leads to a higher blood viscosity, which can impair cerebral blood flow, furthering the damage to the brain. Fluid restriction is not recommended for this type of hyponatremia as it has been associated with increased cerebral infarction. In patients with severe, symptomatic cerebral edema, a hypertonic saline solution may be instituted. A solution of 3% hypertonic saline at a rate of 75 cc/hr should be started. When hypertonic saline is in use, electrolytes should be monitored at a minimum of every 2 hours. Serum sodium and osmolarity should be monitored more frequently, every hour until stabilized, and the hypertonic saline infusion should be titrated to achieve serum sodium 145–155 meq/L and serum osmolarity of 300–320 mOsm/L. Serum potassium should be monitored and replaced to maintain normal levels (3.5–5 mEq/L). Hypertonic saline solutions should be tapered slowly when cerebral edema has resolved and/or if serum sodium rises above 155 meq/L.

Cerebral edema
Cerebral edema occurs for a variety of reasons after neurosurgical procedures. After aneurysmal subarachnoid hemorrhage, the most common cause is hyponatremia that leads to a hypo-osmolar state and blood brain barrier alterations promoting fluid movement into cells and neurons in particular. As water is absorbed into cells of the central nervous system, they stop functioning properly. The increase in cell size leads to an increase in mass inside the cranial vault and, if not treated, can result in increased intracranial pressure and herniation. Cerebral edema is commonly identified by neurologic changes identified during examination. Any change in neurologic functioning warrants additional testing including CT scan and, in some instances, MRI. Flair imaging is helpful in identifying the subtle changes that occur in the face of cerebral edema. When cerebral edema develops, hypertonic saline should be used as a first-line treatment. A 2–3% solution at a rate of 75–100 cc/hr should be administered unless contraindicated. Electrolytes including serum sodium and potassium should be assessed at a minimum of every 6 hours, but more frequently when the infusion is initiated, after the dose has been changed, or with development of any new deficits. Potassium should be replaced as necessary to maintain levels within normal limits. The infusion should be titrated to maintain serum sodium within the range of 145–155 mEq/L and serum osmolarity at 300–320 mOsm/L. Once cerebral edema has resolved, hypertonic saline infusion should be tapered off. Hypertonic saline should only be used as long as clinically warranted, as the potential side effects of excess dosing are lethal.

Respiratory

Patients recovering from SAH have varying needs for respiratory support. Continuous pulse oximetry monitoring should be employed to monitor for adequate oxygenation and potential change in status. The pulse oximeter alarm should be set to alert at a saturation of 89%, and the goal of treatment should be to maintain oxygen saturation at or above 90%. Patients with cardiac or pulmonary comorbidities may need higher goals.

For the patient who is not having difficulty maintaining his/her airway and has adequate oxygen saturation by pulse oximeter or arterial blood gases, no treatment may be necessary. For patients who have oxygen saturation less than 90%, oxygen therapy should be initiated. The minimum amount of oxygen necessary to maintain the goal of 90% or higher saturation via pulse oximeter should be administered in the least invasive manner possible.

Acute lung impairment and respiratory distress syndrome are common in the SAH population. For the patient who is not able to maintain his/her airway or those without proper oxygenation, using external oxygen administration devices (nasal cannula, face mask), intubation, and mechanical ventilation are necessary. Ventilator settings should provide adequate oxygenation to maintain arterial blood gas, pulse oximeter, and (if used) end tidal CO_2 values (≥ 37 mmHg) within normal limits. PEEP has been shown to be safe and effective in aSAH patients and may be used as needed (Caricato et al., 2005), although it is important to monitor blood pressure and cerebral perfusion in this instance. Suctioning to clear secretions should be administered as needed. Pre-suctioning hyperoxygenation (100% O_2) is recommended. Saline lavage pre-suctioning should be avoided as it promotes decreased oxygenation and infection. Suctioning should be performed for less than 15 seconds with breaks allowing the return of oxygen saturation to normal levels in between attempts.

Cardiac

Blood pressure goals

Sympathetic activation immediately after SAH causes significant increase in blood pressure in many patients. This may be exacerbated by anxiety and/or pain in patients who are not comatose.

Blood pressure management

a. Analgesia

Pain and anxiety are significant problems for the patient recovering from SAH. The increase in mass within the cranial vault leads to increases in intracranial pressure that can cause headache/pain. Sympathetic activation may be perceived as anxiety. Further, psychological distress may occur due to a traumatic, emergent situation and lead to anxiety presenting as an increase in blood pressure and heart rate, among other symptoms. Treatment of pain with analgesics often decreases pain and sympathetic response and relieves anxiety, bringing blood pressure within the target range.

Acetaminophen has been shown to provide adequate relief of pain in some patients. For those not receiving adequate relief, narcotic analgesia is likely required. Acetaminophen with codeine or other narcotic analgesics may be used as needed to provide adequate relief to the majority of patients with SAH. For those whose pain persists beyond this threshold, fentanyl or other intravenous sedative/analgesic may be warranted.

Regardless of which medication is used for pain relief, the smallest dose achieving efficacy should be used. This is particularly true when narcotics are being used which induce decreased level of consciousness and can mask neurologic changes signaling a more severe neurologic problem such as rebleed, hydrocephalus, seizures, cerebral vasospasm, delayed cerebral ischemia, stroke, or meningitis.

b. Vasoactive medications

In many instances, analgesia will relieve pain and anxiety without bringing blood pressure within the target range. In these instances, additional vasoactive medications are required. The goal of blood pressure is to support oxygen and nutrient delivery to brain tissue, which is best achieved when CPP is above 60 mmHg. This may be achieved by modifying blood pressure and/or controlling intracranial pressure. For guidelines on intracranial pressure management, see page 111. Systolic blood pressure should be maintained between 90 and 140 mmHg.

Patients with an elevated MAP may have low CPP despite normal ICP. If a patient has a MAP greater than 140, assuming an ICP of 20 mmHg, CPP is 120 and hyperemia may occur. Once the AVM or aneurysm is secured, rebleed is not an issue and blood pressure above 140 mmHg may occur. Systolic blood pressure up to 200 mmHg is acceptable. While not commonly needed, agents to maintain systolic blood pressure at less than 200 mmHg are occasionally required.

For patients with low MAP, the primary risk is inadequate cerebral perfusion, hypoxia, ischemia, and stroke. Blood pressure may be increased with fluid volume (see the next subsection) and a variety of medications may be used.

c. Fluid balance

A decrease in blood pressure in any patient in the ICU may be related to decreased fluid volume. In patients with central venous pressure (CVP) monitoring, fluids should be administered to maintain CVP 5–8 mmHg, a euvolemic state. While the administration of normal saline solution (0.9% NaCL) at 100 cc/hr will generally maintain a euvolemic state, intravenous boluses of 250 cc normal saline may be administered. It is generally not recommended to administer multiple boluses of normal saline as this may induce hemodilution. For patients experiencing cerebral vasospasm/DCI, additional fluid may be needed to maintain adequate perfusion and a CVP 8–12 mmHg. See page 114–118 for specific guidelines for treatment of patients with cerebral vasospasm and DCI.

Other support and prevention

a. Gastrointestinal

Nutrition should be provided in the most independent way possible. For patients who are alert and without swallowing problems, a normal diet should be provided. Some assessment of the swallowing function by personnel trained in this area should occur before food or fluids are provided. Many facilities use speech therapists to perform this assessment, while others utilize nurses. Some patients are able to swallow solids without incidence but have issues with liquids, and liquid thickeners should be used to prevent aspiration. For patients not able to tolerate their regular diet, a soft diet may be warranted. For patients not able to eat any diet due to coma or tracheotomy, enteral nutrition should be provided if tolerated. There are many formulas for enteral feeding and the decision should be guided by the patient's nutritional needs and medical conditions. For patients with renal or liver disease, special formulas are available and should be utilized. A small number of patients recovering from SAH may have gastrointestinal problems that prohibit enteral feedings. In these select patients, parenteral nutrition should be provided. Again, the selection of the specific formula of parenteral nutrition should be based on individual patient's medical conditions and nutritional needs.

Stress ulcers are a common occurrence in critically ill patients. Some form of ulcer prophylaxis should be initiated. H_2 antagonists, cytoprotective agents, and proton pump inhibitors all provide adequate coverage. Stress ulcer prophylaxis should be provided during the entire intensive care unit stay and prolonged use in the step-down, general unit and after discharge should be considered based on individual patient's medical status, other medications, and symptoms.

Elimination should be assessed on a regular basis and treatment should be provided to promote bowel movements of consistency and frequency the patient experienced before admission. Many medications can cause constipation or diarrhea. Docusate sodium may be given prophylactically to maintain soft stool in any patient but is particularly helpful in those taking constipating narcotics or with limited mobility. A variety of other medications can be used to maintain proper elimination without inducing new neurologic injury or deficit.

b. Integumentary

Patients recovering from subarachnoid hemorrhage often are on bed rest in the very acute period. In patients who are awake and alert, the risk of skin breakdown, often known as bedsores, is not significantly high. They are generally able to move themselves around in bed to prevent prolonged pressure on specific areas. Patients who are awake, alert, and capable of moving should be encouraged to move around in bed and turn frequently (every few hours) to prevent skin breakdown.

In patients who are comatose due to the hemorrhage or medications, the risk of skin breakdown is higher. They are not able to spontaneously move and alleviate pressure points. It is important to turn these patients every 2 hours to prevent skin breakdown. An alternating schedule outlining time on each side and back is helpful to maintain turning across shifts.

Other general measures to maintain intact skin include providing proper nutrition, daily bathing with more frequent washing of areas that become soiled, and keeping skin hydrated but dry. The period of time a patient is on strict bed rest should be limited to prevent skin breakdown and promote musculoskeletal health.

c. Musculoskeletal

Patients in the intensive care unit often have limited mobility for a variety of reasons. Medications, ventilation, pain, and hemodynamic instability often hamper efforts to move the patient in bed and get the patient out of bed. A consult to physical therapist and occupational therapist should occur soon after admission, even for unconscious patients. There is no evidence specific to the subarachnoid hemorrhage population, but evidence from a general ICU population suggests that early mobility promotes gastrointestinal function in addition to limiting musculoskeletal problems induced by bed rest. It is advised that the maximum level of musculoskeletal functioning should be provided or encouraged as early as possible while maintaining patient safety. In the very acute period of 1–2 days, bed rest should be maintained and a range of motion should be performed or encouraged frequently. If the patient is able to move, an active range of motion should be encouraged by the nurse every 2 hours. Patients who are comatose or heavily sedated require a passive range of motion provided by the nurse, physical therapist, or other trained staff member every 2 hours. Patients recovering from subarachnoid hemorrhage should get out of bed in the first few days. If they are able, walking the halls of the intensive care unit with assistance or observation is ideal. It is important to have adequate staff available to walk with the patient, monitoring for steadiness and assuring drains and catheters remain intact. Measures should be taken to ensure the patient is safe and does not walk to the point of exhaustion. It is recommended that a staff member walk alongside the patient providing support of the patient and drains, catheters, IV poles, and so forth, and an additional staff member walk behind the patient with a wheelchair in the event the patient becomes exhausted or has hemodynamic instability.

For patients who are not able to walk due to low level of consciousness, hemodynamic instability, or other injury impairing mobility, getting out of bed to a chair should occur at least twice a day and more frequently as tolerated. Patients sitting out of bed should not be left for more than two hours without repositioning to prevent skin breakdown.

Once transferred out of the intensive care unit, the patient should be encouraged to spend as much time out of bed as possible and walk frequently and independently if possible. Comatose patients still require significant and frequent range of motion exercises and time sitting in chairs.

LONG-TERM CARE

Patients with subarachnoid hemorrhage have long-term needs similar to those of patients with other stroke subtypes, and individual patient's needs, family abilities and resources, and financial/ insurance requirements need to be considered. Once the patient is stable enough for discharge from the hospital, many settings may be considered. The setting that provides the highest level of independence while maintaining safety and continued recovery should be selected. There are no clear guidelines for discharge specific to patients recovering from subarachnoid hemorrhage. If the patient is able to carry out activities of daily living and has support at home, discharge to home is ideal. Outpatient rehabilitation should be considered and is often necessary for these patients. In addition to physical rehabilitation, it is important to consider cognitive functioning and the potential need for cognitive therapy. This should be evaluated at subsequent follow-up visits to promote maximum physical and cognitive recovery for the patient recovering from subarachnoid hemorrhage. Patients with significant physical or cognitive deficits who are awake and able to move around but not quite stable or independent enough for discharge to home may be referred to inpatient rehabilitation settings. Some patients recovering from subarachnoid hemorrhage will not be physically or cognitively able to participate in rehabilitation and may need to spend time in other, higher level of care settings until discharge to a rehabilitation setting or home. Some patients will require long-term acute care, assisted living, or nursing home care with full support.

Upon discharge from the acute hospital, several things should be considered regardless of discharge disposition. The need for blood pressure management will need to be evaluated. While the patient with a secured aneurysm or AVM is at fairly low risk of rebleed, hypertension should still be treated due to other negative sequelae. General health promotion concepts including diet and exercise should be discussed and a healthy lifestyle promoted. Frequently, patients recovering from subarachnoid hemorrhage need to follow up with the neurosurgical management team in one to three months. A cerebral angiogram should be performed to verify aneurysm securement or AVM obliteration. Repeated visits to the neurosurgical team should occur at 6 months and 1 year to evaluate neurologic functioning and assess the need for rehabilitation services, seizure control medication continuation, and other medications.

REFERENCES
Awad, I. A., Carter, L. P., Spetzler, R. F., Medina, M., & Williams Jr., F. C. (1987). Clinical vasospasm after subarachnoid hemorrhage: Response to hypervolemic hemodilution and arterial hypertension. *Stroke, 18*(2), 365–372.

Caricato, A., Conti, G., Della Corte, F., et al. (2005). Effects of PEEP on the intracranial system of patients with head injury and subarachnoid hemorrhage: The role of respiratory system compliance. *Journal of Trauma-Injury Infection & Critical Care, 58*(3), 571–576.

Claassen, J., Carhuapoma, R., Kreiter, K. T., Du, E. Y., Connolly, E. S., & Mayer, S. A. (2002). Global cerebral edema after subarachnoid hemorrhage: Frequency, predictors, and impact on outcome. *Stroke, 33*(5), 1225–1232.

Clozel, M. (2000). Endothelin receptor antagonists: Current status and perspectives. *Journal of Cardiovascular Pharmacology, 35*(4 Suppl 2), S65–S68.

Cormio, M., & Citerio, G. (2007). Continuous low dose diclofenac sodium infusion to control fever in neurosurgical critical care. *Neurocritical Care, 6*(2), 82–89.

Deibert, E., Barzilai, B., Braverman, A. C., et al. (2003). Clinical significance of elevated troponin I levels in patients with nontraumatic subarachnoid hemorrhage. *Journal of Neurosurgery*, *98*(4), 741–746.

Doczi, T., Bende, J., Huszka, E., & Kiss, J. (1981). Syndrome of inappropriate secretion of antidiuretic hormone after subarachnoid hemorrhage. *Neurosurgery*, *9*(4), 394–397.

Fujii, Y., Takeuchi, S., Sasaki, O., Minakawa, T., Koike, T., & Tanaka R. (1996). Ultra-early rebleeding in spontaneous subarachnoid hemorrhage. *Journal of Neurosurgery*, *84*(1), 35–42.

Fults, D., & Kelly Jr., D. L. (1984). Natural history of arteriovenous malformations of the brain: A clinical study. *Neurosurgery*, *15*(5), 658–662.

Hravnak, M., Frangiskakis, J. M., Crago, E. A., et al. (2009). Elevated cardiac troponin I and relationship to persistence of electrocardiographic and echocardiographic abnormalities after aneurysmal subarachnoid hemorrhage. *Stroke*, *40*(11), 3478–3484.

Janjua, N., & Mayer, S. A. (2003). Cerebral vasospasm after subarachnoid hemorrhage. *Current Opinion in Critical Care*, *9*(2), 113–119.

Kassell, N. F., Peerless, S. J., Durward, Q. J., Beck, D. W., Drake, C. G., & Adams, H. P. (1982). Treatment of ischemic deficits from vasospasm with intravascular volume expansion and induced arterial hypertension. *Neurosurgery*, *11*(3), 337–343.

Macdonald, R. L., Higashida, R. T., Keller, E., et al. (2011). Clazosentan, an endothelin receptor antagonist, in patients with aneurysmal subarachnoid haemorrhage undergoing surgical clipping: A randomised, double-blind, placebo-controlled phase 3 trial (CONSCIOUS-2). *Lancet Neurology*, *10*(7), 618–625.

Marinov, M. B., Harbaugh, K. S., Hoopes, P. J., Pikus, H. J., & Harbaugh, R. E. (1996). Neuroprotective effects of preischemia intraarterial magnesium sulfate in reversible focal cerebral ischemia. *Journal of Neurosurgery*, *85*(1), 117–124.

Mayer, S. A., Kowalski, R. G., Presciutti, M., et al. (2004). Clinical trial of a novel surface cooling system for fever control in neurocritical care patients. *Critical Care Medicine*, *32*(12), 2508–2515.

Molyneux, A. J., Kerr, R. S. C., Yu, L.-M., et al. (2005). International subarachnoid aneurysm trial (ISAT) of neurosurgical clipping versus endovascular coiling in 2143 patients with ruptured intracranial aneurysms: A randomised comparison of effects on survival, dependency, seizures, rebleeding, subgroups, and aneurysm occlusion. *Lancet, 366*(9488), 809–817.

Muench, E., Bauhuf, C., Roth, H., et al. (2005). Effects of positive end-expiratory pressure on regional cerebral blood flow, intracranial pressure, and brain tissue oxygenation. *Critical Care Medicine, 33*(10), 2367–2372.

Muizelaar, J. P., & Becker, D. P. (1986). Induced hypertension for the treatment of cerebral ischemia after subarachnoid hemorrhage: Direct effect on cerebral blood flow. *Surgical Neurology, 25*(4), 317–325.

Muroi, C., Terzic, A., Fortunati, M., Yonekawa, Y., & Keller, E. (2008). Magnesium sulfate in the management of patients with aneurysmal subarachnoid hemorrhage: A randomized, placebo-controlled, dose-adapted trial. *Surgical Neurology, 69*(1), 33–39; discussion on p. 39.

Nogueira, R. G., Bodock, M. J., Koroshetz, W. J., et al. (2007). High-dose bosentan in the prevention and treatment of subarachnoid hemorrhage-induced cerebral vasospasm: An open-label feasibility study. *Neurocritical Care, 7*(3), 194–202.

Pyne, G. J., Cadoux-Hudson, T. A., & Clark, J. F. (2001). Magnesium protection against in vitro cerebral vasospasm after subarachnoid haemorrhage. *British Journal of Neurosurgery, 15*(5), 409–415.

Qureshi, A. I., Suri, M. F. K., Sung, G. Y., et al. (2002). Prognostic significance of hypernatremia and hyponatremia among patients with aneurysmal subarachnoid hemorrhage. *Neurosurgery, 50*(4), 749–755; discussion on pp. 749–755.

Ram, Z., Sadeh, M., Shacked, I., Sahar, A., & Hadani, M. (1991). Magnesium sulfate reverses experimental delayed cerebral vasospasm after subarachnoid hemorrhage in rats. *Stroke, 22*(7), 922–927.

Suarez, J. I., Tarr, R. W., & Selman W. R. (2006). Aneurysmal subarachnoid hemorrhage. *New England Journal of Medicine, 354*(4), 387–396.

van den Bergh, W. M., Albrecht, K. W., Berkelbach van der Sprenkel, J. W., & Rinkel, G. J. E. (2003). Magnesium therapy after aneurysmal subarachnoid haemorrhage: A dose-finding study for long-term treatment. *Acta Neurochirurgica, 145*(3), 195–199; discussion on p. 199.

van den Bergh, W. M., van de Water, J. M. W., Hoff, R. G., Algra, A., & Rinkel, G. J. E. (2008). Calcium homeostasis during magnesium treatment in aneurysmal subarachnoid hemorrhage. *Neurocritical Care, 8*(3), 413–417.

van den Bergh, W. M., Zuur, J. K., Kamerling, N. A., et al. (2002). Role of magnesium in the reduction of ischemic depolarization and lesion volume after experimental subarachnoid hemorrhage. *Journal of Neurosurgery, 97*(2), 416–422.

Van der Schaaf, I., Algra, A., Wermer, M. J., et al. (2009). Endovascular coiling versus neurosurgical clipping for patients with aneurysmal subarachnoid haemorrhage. *Cochrane Database Systematic Review, 4*(CD003085).

van Norden, A. G. W., van den Bergh, W. M., Rinkel, G. J. E. (2005). Dose evaluation for long-term magnesium treatment in aneurysmal subarachnoid haemorrhage. *Journal of Clinical Pharmacy & Therapeutics, 30*(5), 439–442.

Veyna, R. S., Seyfried, D., Burke, D. G., et al. (2002). Magnesium sulfate therapy after aneurysmal subarachnoid hemorrhage. *Journal of Neurosurgery, 96*(3), 510–514.

Wartenberg, K. E., & Mayer S. A. (2006). Medical complications after subarachnoid hemorrhage: New strategies for prevention and management. *Current Opinion in Critical Care, 12*(2), 78–84.

Cerebral Amyloid Angiopathy

6

Alice E. Davis

Evidence-Based Nursing Care for Stroke and Neurovascular Conditions,
First Edition. Edited by Sheila A. Alexander.
© 2013 John Wiley & Sons, Inc. Published 2013 by John Wiley & Sons, Inc.

DEFINITION
CAA is an asymptomatic disorder, yet a primary cause of intracerebral hemorrhage in the elderly. By definition, amyloid is an insoluble aggregated protein fragment. The amyloid form is taken on as a result of an alteration in the pattern of hydrogen bonds or what is known as the secondary structure of the protein. Amyloid can be deposited in tissue, organs, or blood vessels. In the case of CAA, congophilic amyloid deposits are found in the capillaries, arterioles, small and medium-sized vessels of the cerebral cortex, cerebellum, and leptomeninges. Distribution is patchy, but there is predominance within the occipital lobe and less in the cerebellum (Greenberg, 2009). Deeper vessels of the white and gray matter are spared. CAA has been identified with a myriad of disorders including Alzhiemer Disease (AD), Down syndrome, post-radiation brain necrosis, and demylenating disorders similar to multiple sclerosis. In severe CAA, microinfarcts have been identified, and there is much speculation of a CAA-induced inflammatory process (Vinters, 1987).

HISTORICAL PERSPECTIVE
CAA was likely identified first by Fisher and Oppenheimer during the early part of the 20th century (Greenberg & Levine, 2010). Although several labels were given to the condition, it was not until 1927, when a congo red stain was applied to tissue and viewed under polarized light, that amyloid deposition was described by Divry as congophilic angiopathy (Greenberg, 2009; Greenberg & Levine, 2010). Vascular amyloid invading brain tissue was termed dysphoric angiopathy later in the middle of the century by Morel and Wildi (Greenberg & Levine, 2010). By the 1940s, both the familial association in Iceland and the link to dementia were reported. CAA became an integral part of AD and was linked to non-traumatic intracerebral hemorrhage by the 1970s. CAA is now considered to be a common pathology in older persons, a significant contributing factor for AD, and a major contributor to intracerebral hemorrhagic stroke (Attems, 2005; Greenberg & Levine, 2010).

EPIDEMIOLOGY
CAA has been identified as a sporadic disorder and has been linked to familial syndromes and early onset of dementia. It is difficult to

ascertain the true incidence and prevalence of CAA, given that a definitive diagnosis of CAA is made at a postmorten examination. The prevalence in older adults has been estimated to be between 10% and 14% and greater than 80% in those with AD. The presence of epsilon4 allele of apolipoprotein E (ApoE) and ApoE-2 is a risk factor for CAA, but only ApoE-2 increases the risk for hemorrhage in CAA. Based on autopsy evidence of patients who died following a lobar intracerebral hemorrhage (ICH), CAA was found in 18.3% of men and 28% of women aged 40–90. Increasing prevalence with age is well documented, with severity and extent of the pathology steadily increasing over time (Greenberg & Vonsattel, 1997; Pezzini et al., 2009). CAA has not been correlated with common cerebral vascular risk such as hypertension, diabetes, hyperlipidemia, or arthrosclerosis (Yamada, 2000; Greenberg, 2009).

Many subtypes of CAA have been identified and are presented in Table 6.1. The sporadic form of CAA is the most common type and is found in the brains of elderly persons with or without AD. There are documented familial forms that occur at a younger age; these include Icelandic, Dutch, British, and Finnish types. In addition, there has been a familial amyloid angiopathy associated with deafness and ocular hemorrhage (Yamada, 2000; Thanvi & Robinson, 2006).

PATHOPHYSIOLOGY

CAA is a progressive disorder; its hallmark deposition of amyloid has been identified in live and postmortem brains. It has been found in the cerebral vascular walls in aging persons with and without AD pathology. A simple explanation for CAA is unlikely. Both pathogenetic and biomolecular events are at play in the development of Abeta and subsequent CAA. The extent and interaction of genetic and biomolecular events are not clear, as evidenced by the identification of CAA in brains of normal aging individuals, those with AD, and those with specific familial genetic markers.

Although several cerebrovascular amyloid proteins have been identified, Abeta is most readily associated with sporadic and hereditary forms of CAA (Yamada, 2000). The amyloid beta-peptide is a 39-43 amino acid fragment of the amyloid precursor protein (APP). The fragment Abeta is a neurotoxic chemical that results from the catabolism of the APP. Mutations of the APP encoding

Table 6.1 Types, proteins, features, and characteristics of CAA

Types	Protein	Features	Characteristics
Sporadic CAA CAA of Abeta	Abeta		ICH, infarction, vaculitis, vascular malformations, microbleeds, inflammation, cognitive decline, AD pathology, Down Syndrome, normal aging
HCDWA-DHCHWA-It	Aabtae	Autosomal dominant disorder of Dutch families	Occurs in middle age, with recurrent lobar cerebral hemorrhages and leukoencephalopathy
HCDWA-I	Cystatin C (ACys) in CSF	Autosomal dominant disorder of Icelandic families	Causes severe CAA with recurrent cerebral hemorrhages before age 40
Prion Protein (PrP)-Japanese	PrP (Ascr) type	Japanese patient with progressive dementia	PrP deposits found with Neuro fibrillatory tangles (NFT); no hemorrhage
ABr (A-WD)	ABr-novel 4K protein subunit in isolated amyloid fibrils	Autosomal dominant disorder of British families	Progressive spastic paralysis, dementia, ataxia, severe CAA, NFT, non-neuritic and perivascular plaques, ischemic leukoencephalopathy
Hereditary amyloidoses of Transthyretin (TTR) (prealbumin) type	ATTR; TRR is produced in the choroid plexus and liver	Autosomal dominant mutations of the TTR gene; seen in Japan, Portugal and other countries; associated with FAP type 1; TTR amylodoses w different TRR mutations	Peripheral and autonomic neuropathies alone; leptomeningeal and meningovascular amyloid deposits with hemorrhage, infarction, hydrocephalus, oculoleptomeningeal amyloidosis, paresis, and dementia.
Gelsolin (AGel) type: familial amyloidosis, Finnish type	Mutation	Rare disorder of Finnish relatives carrying G654A or G654T mutations	Facial palsy, mild peripheral neuropathies, spinal, cerebral and meningeal amyloid angiopathy associated with white matter lesions

HCDWA-D – hereditary cerebral hemorrhage with amyloidosis Dutch-type
HCDWA-It – hereditary cerebral hemorrhage with amyloidosis Italian-type
HCDWA-I – hereditary cerebral hemorrhage with amyloidosis Icelandic-type
ABr (A-WD) – British or Worster-Drought type
FAP – familial amyloid polyneuropathy
Adapted from Yamada (2000).

gene have been identified as responsible for some cases of presenile CAA. Other evidence supports APP mutations, especially in the familial types of CAA that increases toxicity to the vessel walls. Still other work suggests a mutational effect on the ability of Abeta proteolysis or clearance from the CNS (Tsubuki, Takaki, & Saido, 2003; Davis et al., 2004; Obici et al., 2005).

The Abeta accumulation begins with amyloid deposits at the border of cerebral vessels along the media and adventia. The Abeta decreases the width but increases the size of the vessel and damages the muscular lamina, rendering the vessel rigid and fragile (Bugiani, 2004). In advanced forms of CAA, there is loss of vascular smooth muscle, resulting in vasculopathic changes such as microaneurysms with dilation, double-barrel lumens, intimal lining changes, hyaline degeneration, chronic perivascular inflammation, and fibrinoid necrosis. These changes have been associated with leakage of blood products laying the foundation for symptomatic CAA related hemorrhages (Yamada, 2000; Greenberg, 2009).

The use of animal models has aided in the understanding of Abeta elimination from the brain. According to these models, Abeta is moved either directly from the brain to the blood or along perivascular interstitial fluid channels. Preston et al. (2003) reported that Abeta elimination along the perivascular channels enters the pericapillary spaces into the cortical arteries and then to the leptomeningeal arteries. The results of this study suggest that when Abeta is eliminated from the extracellular spaces of the human brain by the perivascular route, it enters pericapillary spaces and then drains along the walls of cortical arteries to leptomeningeal arteries. The researchers hypothesized that overproduction, entrapment, or poor drainage might slow elimination, contributing to the accumulation of Abeta in the cerebral and leptomeningeal arteries (Preston et al., 2003).

Accumulation of Abeta in the cerebral vasculature has lead researchers to examine issues related to production, clearance, and aggregation (Davis et al., 2004; Bateman et al., 2007; Mawuenyega et al., 2010). Neurons, cerebrovascular cells, or the circulation itself may be the source of the Abeta deposited along or across the vessel walls with accumulation in the extracellular spaces caused by several mutations in the Abeta precursor and presenlin genes (Rensink, de Waal, Kremer, & Verbeek, 2003). Similar accumulation of Abeta in cerebral vessels and extracellular spaces occurs as a part of normal aging (Love et al., 2009). Therefore, the distribution and pathogenicity of Abeta has been linked to degradation of paranchymal and vascular Abeta and production of Abeta in the perivascular extracellular matrix (Love et al., 2009). Several hypotheses are offered to explain the Abeta vascular deposition, including an increase in Abeta 40 and Abeta 42, an impedance of perivascular passage of Abeta, or a rise in the concentration of Abeta, which may or may not be related to a reduction in Abeta degrading enzymes (Love et al., 2009).

DIAGNOSIS

The diagnosis of CAA is based on a number of factors including clinical criteria, diagnostic imaging, and newly emerging biomarkers.

Clinical diagnostic criteria

The Boston criteria, a standardized set of diagnostic criteria for CAA-related hemorrhage, were proposed by a group of neurologists known as the Boston Cerebral Amyloid Angiopathy Group in 1995. The criteria provide a combination of clinical, radiological, and pathological data to categorize CAA. The four levels of certainty proposed and validated were definite, probable with supporting pathological evidence, probable, and possible (Table 6.2) (Smith & Greenberg, 2003).

In addition to the categorization of CAA set forth by the Boston criteria, clinical manifestations of CAA have also been documented (Kumar-Singh, 2008). These features of CAA are listed in Table 6.3.

Neuroimaging

Serial Magnetic Resonance Imaging (MRI): MRI reveals the dynamic and evolving nature of CAA and is used as a diagnostic and prognostic tool. MRI has validated CAA as a subclinical yet progressive disease (Menon & Kidwell, 2009). Findings on MRI demonstrate multiple cortical and subcortical small-to-large hemorrhages even in patients without a history of hemorrhage. These silent hemorrhages in asymptomatic patients may be a marker of disease progression. In gradient-echo sequences of the MRI, hemosiderin deposition corresponding to old hemorrhages has been found. Hemosiderin, derived from hemoglobin, is a result

Table 6.2 Boston criteria for diagnosis of CAA

Definite CAA
Based on full post-mortem examination

  Hemorrhage in lobar, cortical, or cortical areas
  Severe CAA evidenced by pathological evidence of vasculopathy

Probable CAA as supported with pathological evidence

Clinical data and pathological tissue (evacuated hematoma or cortical biopsy specimen) demonstrate

  Lobar, cortical, or cortico/subcortical hemorrhage
  Amyloid deposition to some degree in specimen
  No other diagnostic explanations for hemorrhage

Probable CAA
Clinical and Imaging Support w/o pathological confirmation

  Patient 55 years of age or older
  Clinical history
  Multiple hemorrhages of lobar, cortical, subcortical, or cerebellar area per
MRI/CT

  No other diagnostic explanations for hemorrhage

Possible CAA

  Patient 55 years of age or older
  Single hemorrhage of lobar, cortical, or subcortical areas per MRI/CT
  Supporting clinical history
  No other diagnostic explanations for hemorrhage

Adapted from: Chao et al. (2006); Greenberg & Vonsattel (1997); Knudsen, Rosand, Karluk, et al. (2001); Smith & Greenberg (2003).

Table 6.3 Clinical Manifestations of CAA

Primary Intracranial Hemorrhage
Progressive Cognitive Decline
Cerebral Ischemia and Infarction
Perivascular Inflammation
Leukoencephalopathy
Microbleeds on MRI
Dementia

Created from information found in Kumar-Singh (2008).

of red cell breakdown; it is a yellow-brown protein found in body tissue and phagocytes. Microbleeds of the white matter may also be found, suggesting hemorrhage-prone vasculopathy. The presence of asymptomatic microbleeds raises concerns over the use of thrombolytic, anticoagulant, or antiplatelet therapies.

The use of positron emission tomography (PET) scanning is still emerging. However, there has been an association between increased uptake of 11C-Pittsburgh compound B (PIB), a ligand that binds to beta-amyloid, and patients with CAA-related hemorrhage (Ly et al., 2010). Other imaging modalities used to a much lesser extent are computed tomography (CT) for documentation of intracerebral hemorrhage and angiography.

Biomarkers

Slower clearance of Abeta in the CSF was reported by Bateman et al. (2006), suggesting the accumulation of Abeta was related to dysfunctional clearing mechanisms, not overproduction. Later, Abeta 40 and 42 in CSF suggested trapping of 40 and 42 (isoforms of Abeta that aggregate) in cerebral vasculature from interstitial fluid pathways that transport Abeta proteins to CSF (Verbeek et al., 2009). The use of CSF to determine Abeta levels is thought to be the first step in the development of a biomarker for Abeta. Efforts to establish a serum CAA biomarker are ongoing (Bateman, Munsella, et al., 2006; Bateman, Wen, et al., 2007; Verbeek et al., 2009; Blennow et al., 2010).

Other diagnostic considerations

Microhemorrhage-multiple microhemorrhages or microbleeds found on MRI are part of the diagnostic criteria for CAA. However, a single focus alone may not be solely attributed to CAA, as these can be attributed to other amyloid related causes such as hypertensive microangiopathy or endocarditis (Klein et al., 2009). From a prognostic perspective, the number of recurrent microbleeds has been associated with increasing risk for primary lobar hemorrhage. In addition, microbleeds were predictive of higher risk for of cognitive impairment, loss of functional independence, stroke, and death (Greenberg et al., 2004; Altmann-Schneider et al., 2011).

Issue Examination – As part of routine examination, excised tissue, including hematomas and cortical and leptomeningeal tissue, should be stained with Congo red and examined for CAA. Presence of CAA in these tissues suggests advanced disease and indicates that these patients are at risk for hemorrhage (Greenberg & Kasner, 2011). In postmortem review of CAA, related hemorrhage tissue demonstrated the characteristics of varying degrees of CAA disease, including complete replacement of the muscle layer of the vessel or evidence of vessel breakdown (Mandybur, 1986; Greenberg & Vonsattel, 1997).

Other testing

Laboratory studies evaluating coagulation status such as pro-thrombin, activated partial thromboplastin time, and platelet count should be performed. In view of the potential risk for intracerebral hemorrhage in patients with CAA, these tests can identify CAA patients with bleeding disorders that need to be addressed. Analysis of CSF for detection of changing levels of Abeta 40 and 42 and increased levels of tau have the potential of distinguishing CAA patients (Verbeek et al., 2009).

Associated diagnoses

CAA has been linked to or known to cause numerous other syndromes in addition to AD. These syndromes are discussed below and include: microvascular ischemia and infarction, asymptomatic microbleeds, white matter changes such as leukoencephalopathy, cognitive impairment, and CAA inflammation (Yamada, 2000; Rensink et al., 2003).

Cortical ischemia and microinfarcts

The deposition of amyloid protein, responsible for CAA, is considered a major cause of microvascular ischemic disease and lobar cerebral and cerebellar hemorrhages and small vessel cortical infarct and hemorrhages in older adults (Yamada, 2000). Advanced CAA was reported in a significant proportion of vascular dementia cases by Haglund et al. (2006), suggesting a CAA-related vascular dementia subtype.

Leukoencephalopathy

Characterized by the destruction of the myelin sheath, leukoencephalopathy was identified in postmortem examinations following lobar hemorrhage. Disease was found in both hemispheres with a diffuse white matter pattern, and was predominant in the periventricular areas (Gray, Dubas, Roullet, & Escourolle, 1985).

CAA microbleeds

CAA is suspected when lobar cerebral microbleeds (CMB) are detected on MRI. CMBs, a neuroimaging finding, are receiving increased attention in dementia, cerebrovascular disease, and normal aging. Specifically, the gradient echo or T2 weighted MRI detects remnants of hemorrhage described as 2–5 mm focal or multifocal areas of hemosiderin (Greenberg, 2011).

CMBs are a manifestation of small vessel pathology detected on MRI and described as small perivascular hemorrhages (Greenberg et al., 2009; Werring, Gregoire, & Cipolotti, 2010). CAA-related CMBs are highly associated with cognitive decline and suspected to have an indirect effect on cognition through chronic hypoperfusion or neuronal degeneration (Viswanathan et al., 2008). There is evidence that CMBs may have occipital predominance along with parietooccipital leukoaraiosis (diffuse abnormalities of the white matter) and be related to cerebrovascular disease. The evidence for a connection between CAA and leukoaraiosis has been speculated but not firmly established (Petterson et al., 2008). CMBs are thought to be important clinical features and, if found early, may identify persons at risk for ICH.

Cognitive impairment

The association between AD and CAA has been well established; however, CAA has also been implicated with other forms of cognitive dysfunction. Greenberg, Edip-Gurol, Rosand, and Smith (2004) compared cognitive function during life with autopsy results and determined CAA was an independent risk factor for cognitive dysfunction after controlling for both age and AD pathology. Cognitive impairment was also associated with the white matter changes demonstrated in imaging studies performed on patients with CAA-related ICH (Greenberg et al., 2004). There is also speculation that a combination of CAA and cerebrovascular disease (CVD) may be a cause of dementia alone or may lower the threshold for AD-like

Table 6.4 CAA Inflammation (CAAI)

Clinical Features	MRI Results	Laboratory Studies	Biopsy
Acute onset confusion	Mass Lesion	CSF protein	Vascular amyloid deposits with perivascular, intramural or transmural inflammatory changes
Short-term memory loss	Leptomenigeal enhancement	CSF Pleocytosis	
Long-term memory loss	Edema	Xanthochromic CSF (microhemorrhage)	
Impaired concentration	Leukoencephalopathy	ESR Elevated above 100	
Visual field deficits		CRP elevated	Multinucleated giant cells
Headache		APOE e4/e4 positive	
Seizures			
Balance problems			
Gait Problems Mono or hemiparesis			

CRP – C-reactive protein
CSF – Cerebral spinal fluid
Created from information found in Chung et al. (2011); Kinnecom et al. (2007).

changes, because patients with CAA/CVD have a higher level of cognitive impairment than AD patients alone (Rensick et al., 2003).

CAA inflammation

CAA inflammation (CAAI) is being increasingly recognized as a subtype of CAA having distinct clinical, pathological, and radiographic features (Table 6.4). Although a less common form of CAA, CAAI has many names including primary angitits of the CNS, amyloid angiopathy, granulomatous angitis of the CNS, cerebral amyloid inflammatory vasculopathy, cerebral amyloid angitis, cerebral amyloid angiopathy associated with giant cell arteritis, and amyloid β-related angitis. Regardless of name, all of these syndromes describe the association between CAA and blood vessel inflammation (Chung et al., 2011). Development of the abnormality has been strongly associated with the ApoE e4/e4 genotype (Kinnecom et al., 2007; Kloppenborg et al., 2010).

CAAI has been described as a subacute progressive encephalopathy. Clinically it has been associated with encephalopathy, acute or subacute headaches, cognitive dysfunction, behavioral changes, focal neurological deficits, and seizures. MRI images demonstrate vasogenic edema and or leukoencephalopathy mimicking space-occupying lesions (Kinnecom et al., 2007; Kloppenborg et al., 2010; Chung et al., 2011).

Two subtypes of CAA have been identified. They can occur alone or together and have similar clinical and imaging features. The non-vasculitic form, also called perivascular infiltration, is characterized by perivascular infiltration of giant cells. The vasculitic form, or transmural (non)-granulomatous angitis, is characterized by inflammation of the vessel wall and is associated with the presence of granulomas (Kinnecom et al., 2007; Kloppenborg et al., 2010). There is histologic evidence that Abeta may be a trigger for the inflammation, because amyloid filled vessels with Abeta are seen in close proximity to the inflamed cells.

Diagnosis

Use of MRI has been reported most often in identifying the two subtypes of CAA related inflammation. White matter edema as well as superficial microhemorrhages characteristics of CAAI can be seen on MRI. Brain biopsy is not necessary given the clinical scenario of cognitive decline, headaches, and seizures (Bernstein, Gibbs, & Batjer, 2011).

Treatment

Various treatment methods have been reported to be effective based on clinical presentation, imaging results, and follow-up reports. Choice of therapy is dependent on patient presentation and duration of therapy is dependent on patient response. Medication is the mainstay of treatment in CAAI, with corticosteroids and immuno-suppressive therapy used most frequently. High-dose corticosteroids have yielded good results and should be measured based on clinical improvement of symptoms and radiographic response

(Bernstein et al., 2011). Use of immunosuppressive agents including pulsed cyclophosphamide (alkylating agent), methotrexate (antimetabolite/antifolate) and mycophenolate mofetil (immunosuppressant) has been reported. There is concern for the use of cyclophosphamide in older, more fragile patients. Antibiotic therapy must always be used if there is suspicion for an infectious agent rather than an inflammatory etiology. Relapses can occur with reduction or cessation of therapy. Anticonvulsants should also be considered (Chung et al., 2011).

CAA COMPLICATIONS
Intracerebral Hemorrhage

As noted previously, the deposition of amyloid protein, responsible for CAA, is considered a major cause of microvascular ischemic disease and lobar hemorrhage in older adults. CAA-related ICH is a result of small vessel disease causing vessel rupture. ICH related to CAA is not related to hypertension but has been associated with use of warfarin. Hemorrhage occurs in the small- to medium-sized blood vessels of the brain and leptomeninges as a result of amyloid deposition that renders the vessels fragile and susceptible to fibrinoid necrosis (Rincon & Mayer, 2008). Risk factors for CAA hemorrhage are age, previous intracerebral hemorrhage, evidence of microbleeds, genetic predisposition, Apolipoprotein E, familial association, dementia, and the presence of ApoE-2.

Primary ICH, a spontaneous extravasation of blood into brain tissue, is the most destructive form of stroke. ICH of CAA etiology accounts for 10–34% of primary ICH, 10–15% of first strokes, 10–30% of stroke admissions, and carries a 30–50% 30-day mortality rate (Sacco & Mayer, 1994; Broderick et al., 2007; Rincon & Mayer, 2008). There is a family prevalence for ICH in certain populations and ICH in a first-degree relative is an independent risk factor for both lobar and nonlobar bleeds (Woo et al., 2002; Towfighi et al., 2005).

Hemorrhage location and onset pattern distinguishes CAA-related ICH from hypertensive bleeds. CAA-related hemorrhages occur in the lobar region of the cerebrum, most frequently in the occipital lobe, occasionally in the cerebellum, and often have extension into the subarachnoid space. They occur more frequently at night. In contrast, hypertensive bleeds rupture into the ventricular space and occur during the day (Towfighi et al., 2005; Greenberg & Levine, 2010). Trigger events are hypothesized to be related to anticoagulation, thrombolytic therapy, and antiplatelet agents. There is conjecture that hypertension, which frequently coexists with CAA in older persons, may also be a trigger, but this has not been supported (Rosand, Hylek, O'Donnell, & Greensberg, 2000; McCarron & Nicoll, 2004).

Location, size, and extension of the bleed as well as surrounding edema and anatomical displacements can be determined by non-enhancing CT scan of the brain. These hemorrhages are often multifocal and recurrent.

Just like other types of strokes, neurological changes following CAA-related hemorrhage reflect the lobar location of the event. Hence clinical manifestations reflecting frontal, parietal, and occipital deficits are predominant and congruent with the side of the hemorrhage. These deficits many include a sudden onset of headache, nausea, or vomiting, change in behavior or change in level of consciousness, motor deficits (hemiparesis), difficulty with expression, sensory or perceptual deficits, spatial neglect, visual deficits (including homonymous hemianopsia), inability to perform complex tasks, and other behaviors indicating change from normal.

Onset of signs and symptoms of ICH can be sudden and evolve over minutes to hours, progressing from onset of a focal neurological deficit in an active person to rapid deterioration, seizures, coma, and death. The size and growth of the hematoma and extension of blood into the ventricles are independent predictors of mortality (Davis et al., 2006; Rordorf & McDonald, 2011), but the volume of ICH and admission score on the Glasgow Coma Scale (GCS) are the most powerful predictors of 30-day mortality (Broderick et al., 2007). If neurological deterioration occurs early (within 48 hours after ICH), the prognosis is poor. Use of anticoagulants and co-morbidities also contribute to poorer outcomes.

The overall approach to treatment of ICH is aggressive care targeted at controlling the bleed, evacuating the hematoma or blood from the brain and ventricles when possible, managing complications including blood pressure changes, increased intracranial pressure (ICP)/decreased cerebral perfusion pressure (CPP), and providing supportive care. A summary of the guideline from the American Heart Association/American Stroke Association, Stroke

Council, High Blood Pressure Research Council, and the Quality of Care and Outcomes in Research Interdisciplinary Working Group is presented in Table 6.5 (Broderick et al., 2007).

A dual treatment approach using both medical and surgical interventions is recommended for ICH management (Table 6.6). There is no evidence to support the use of glucocorticoids, including dexamethasone, in the treatment of ICH.

Because the hemorrhage begins to occupy space in the cranial cavity, there is a risk of developing increased intracranial pressure, cerebral ischemia, and tentorial herniation if interventions are not initiated rapidly. Although surgery is not always indicated, a craniotomy is recommended if there is a larger than 3cm cerebellar hemorrhage, potential for brain stem compression, evidence of obstructive hydrocephalus, large lobar hemorrhage, significant mass effect, or deteriorating status (Broderick et al., 2007; Rincon & Mayer, 2008). There is little evidence to support early versus delayed evacuation of hematomas, but surgery using minimally invasive techniques performed within 12 hours of hemorrhage has garnered some supportive evidence, although early surgery is accompanied by a higher risk for rebleed (Broderick et al., 2007).

Outcomes following surgical intervention of CAA-induced ICH are controversial, demonstrating vastly different degrees of mortality and rates for recurrent bleeding following surgery. Results presented by Petridis (2008) suggest there is no contraindication for evacuation of CAA-related ICH, especially in patients younger than 75 years. This optimistic recommendation is based on analysis of a series of patients with surgical removal of ICH, where a recurrent bleed occurred in 22% of patients, with survival in over half of those patients with re-evacuation despite GCS of 3 in some cases. Overall mortality was 16% post-evacuation, with those aged 75 years or older faring worse.

Aggressive treatment during the first 24 hours after ICH is supported (Broderick et al., 2007). There is some evidence to suggest that early initiation of new do-not-resuscitate (DNR) orders contribute to undertreatment of ICH, linking early use of DNR orders with poor patient outcomes independent of patient's clinical condition (Hemphill, Newman, Zhao, & Johnston, 2004). Use of DNR orders for reasons other than cardiac arrest should be avoided, as too early use of DNR may falsely influence predictive models of

Table 6.5 AHA/ASA Guidelines for Management of ICH

Initial Medical Treatment	Admission to ICU
	Management of ICP elevations
	Maintain fluid balance
	Treat temperature elevations
	Manage blood pressure
	Seizure prophylaxis or control
	Consider use of factor VII
Management of Coagulopathies	Heparin-induced ICH
	Administer protamine sulfate
	Warfarin-Induced ICH
	IV Vitamin K
	Replace clotting factors
	Monitoring INR
	Use of prothrombin, Factor IX, Factor VII to normalize INR more rapid and requires less volume than fresh frozen plasma, but risk for thromboembolism is greater
	Thrombolytic therapy-induced ICH
	Replace clotting factors and platelets
Surgical Recommendations	Cerebellar hemorrhage larger than 3 cm with deterioration
	Evacuation of supratentorial clots within 1 cm of lobar surface (routine evacuation of clots within 96 hours is not recommended)
	Ventricular compression due to hydrocephalus or ventricular obstruction
	Stereotactic infusion of urokinase after 72 hours (risk for rebleed and functional outcome not guaranteed)
Antithrombolytic Therapy	Consider risk for arterial or venous thromboembolism; risk for recurrent ICH, patient condition

Created from information found in Broderick, et al. (2007).

Table 6.6 Medical treatment for the patient with ICH

Airway	Intubation – keep pCO_2 30-35 mmHg; hyperventilation not recommended; secretion management as needed
Circulation	Target BP management based on baseline BP, bleed etiology, age, ICP and CPP; avoid highs and lows as these can result in hypoperfusion/ischemia or rebleed respectively; use vasopressors to maintain MAP and CPP; titrate of vasoactive medications needed for BP and CPP control; SBP $\geq$ 180 mmHg or MAP $\geq$ 130 mmHg require intervention with labetalol, esmolol, or nicardipine. Do not reduce SBP $\geq$ 15–30% during first 24 hours. Maintain CVP 5–8 mmHg
Increased ICP	Target ICP is $\leq$ 20 mmHg; positional intervention to reduce ICP-HOB 30 degrees, midline head placement, avoid 90 degree hip flexion; ventriculostomy for CSF drainage; analgesia, sedation, neuromuscular blockade to manage pain, agitation, refractory ICP; hyperosmolar therapy using 20% mannitol or 3% hypertonic saline; ICP pressure monitoring, consider brain tissue oxygenation, keep CPP $\geq$ 60–70; barbiturate therapy not first-line therapy
Fluid and electrolyte	Maintain euvolemia using isotonic fluids, do not give free water or dextrose solutions; replace electrolytes as needed; especially monitor serum osmolality if using hyperosmolar therapy
DVT and PE prophylaxis	Pneumatic compression devices are recommended, vena cava filters should be considered; consider low-dose heparin after cessation of bleeding; long-term use of antithrombotic therapy for associated conditions (atrial fib) requires evaluation of risk for rebleed, especially in presence of CAA
rFVIIa	Consider within 3–4 hours of bleed to slow progression, but treatment efficacy and safety is not substantiated
Glucose Level	Control hyperglycemia and hypoglycemia episodes; hyperglycemia may be related to preexisting diabetes or acute stress response; judicious lowering is recommended; use of insulin for glucose > 140 mg/dL
Fever	Aggressive treatment of fever is recommended using antipyretic therapy such as acetaminophen; consider complications when using therapeutic cooling
Anticoagulation	Seizure prevention and management using antiepilectic agents such as lorazepam followed by loading dose of phenytoin or fosphenytoin is recommended
Nutrition	Begin enteral feedings with 48 hours using a small-bore nasoduodenal feeding tube

Created from information found in Broderick, et al. (2007); Rincon & Mayer (2008).

Table 6.7 Nursing Care and Monitoring Following ICH

Neurological	Neuro checks q1 and PRN
	Continuous ICP and CPP monitoring
	GCS q 1 hr
	NIHSS on admission and PRN
	Signs and symptoms of hydrocephalus
Cardiovascular	Continuous BP and MAP monitoring
	Arterial line preferred
Fluid & Electrolytes	Monitor I and O
	Monitor electrolytes including Na, K, Mg, Phos, Cl, Ca
	Keep serum osmolality 300–320mOsm/kg
Respiratory	Monitor RR and Rhythm if not intubated
	Pulse Ox keep O_2 Sat > 92%
	Blood gas analysis PRN
	Prevent hypocapnia and hypoxemia
	Prevent aspiration
	Secretion management
Gastrointestinal	Enteral nutrition
	Bowel regimen
Genitourinary	Urine analysis and culture if indicated
Integumentary	Prevent skin breakdown
Muskuloskeletal	Range of motion
	Physical therapy

Courtesy of the National Insitutes of Health National Institute of Neurological Disorders and Stroke.

ICH care and lead to premature withdrawal of treatment during the early stages after the hemorrhage (Hemphill et al., 2004; Broderick et al., 2007).

Nursing care is the mainstay of treatment and is geared toward recognizing the changes associated with increased ICP while monitoring for the adverse effects of the ICH itself and preventing systemic complications. Nursing care is outlined in Table 6.7.

Because of the high morbidity and mortality rates associated with ICH, preventing reoccurrence of ICH is necessary. It is especially important in CAA-related ICH because reoccurrence has been linked both to sporadic and genetically occurring disease. The major risk factors for CAA-related ICH – age and ApoE – are not modifiable; therefore, reduction of associated risk factors including hypertension, smoking, and alcohol use is necessary. Patients who demonstrate evidence of nonlobar microbleeds on MRI without blood pressure elevation should be considered for hypertensive management. Clinical trials using medications that interfere with amyloid deposition on the basement membranes of vessels have been identified but not substantiated (Greenberg, Schneider, & Pettigrew, 2004).

Rehabilitation is considered for all patients upon admission to the hospital and commences once the patient is considered stable. Although rehabilitative care is geared toward promoting ability and independent activity following an ICH, a focus on preventing further disability starts in the acute care setting. Prevention includes turning and positioning to prevent skin breakdown and pressure wounds, consulting a physical therapist to provide range-of-motion activities, and equipment to prevent foot drop and contractures. Use of a speech therapist to evaluate cognitive, swallowing, and speech disorders and an occupational therapist to recommend a plan for resuming activities of daily living is a part of inpatient acute rehabilitative care. Continuation of rehabilitation may be recommended when the patient is deemed ready for discharge from the acute care facility. Further rehabilitation may be performed on an outpatient basis. More likely, older adults will require treatment in either subacute or inpatient rehabilitation facilities. Each of these venues provides rehabilitative care focusing primarily on motor deficits, but the duration and intensity of each program vary. Inpatient rehabilitation is typically the most demanding and requires substantive evaluation by a physiatrist that a patient is ready for the demanding therapy and favorable outcomes can be achieved.

Typical care planning for post-acute care needs following ICH is done with the family and patient if capable. Planning focuses on short-term goals such as the need for further rehabilitation and long-term goals related to independent or assisted living versus continuous support and supervision. A frank discussion of advanced directives should be included in any discussions with an alert patient. The patient's plans for advanced directives including DNR orders as well as wishes for withdrawal of care should be discussed and documented.

RELATED ISSUES IN CAA

Numerous issues have emerged in the recognition and treatment of CAA. These include the use of antithrombotic therapy, management of hypertension, and the progress of medical therapeutics. The section below addresses these concerns.

Use of antithrombotic agents

Lobar ICH, the hallmark of CAA hemorrhage, has been associated with previous microbleeds and has a greater risk for recurrence. Antiplatelet therapy (aspirin) was found to increase the hazard risk (HR) for lobar ICH reoccurrence in all patients whether there was no previous microbleed (HR 1.9) or whether there were up to five previous microbleeds (HR 5.3) (Biffi et al., 2010). It is recommended that caution be taken when using antiplatelet therapy in patients with CAA who have concurrent risk for ischemia related to cerebrovascular or cardiovascular disease (Biffi et al., 2010). Caution is also advised when using nonsteroidal anti-inflammatory medications (Greenberg, 2011).

Anticoagulation therapy

In-vitro reports of Abeta accumulation identify damage to vessel walls causing degeneration, decreased vasoreactivity, and increased proteolytic mechanisms including fibrinolysis, anticoagulation, and degradation of the extracellular matrix (McCarron & Nicoll, 2004). CAA is a frequent cause of warfarin-associated intracerebral hemorrhage. There are also reports linking the use of warfarin with CAA and ICH. Warfarin use in CAA patients was associated with an increase in both frequency and severity of hemorrhage. Thus, warfarin use in this population should be avoided (Greenberg, 2011).

Hypertension

There is no pathological link between CAA and ICH; however, keeping blood pressure within normal limits is advocated. In a secondary analysis of data from the PROGRESS trial, the combined use of Perindopril and ACE inhibitor and indapamide (diuretic) resulted in a 77% reduction of CAA-related ICH (Arima et al., 2010).

DRUG RESEARCH AND DEVELOPMENT

Most of the current drug research focuses on Abeta related to AD. The effect of Abeta is pervasive, leading to the destruction of brain tissue and cerebral blood vessels. Medications under investigation that target Abeta are focusing on decreasing Abeta production, preventing Abeta aggregation, increasing the removal of Abeta, and prophylaxis measures. However, the primary investigations are centered on reduction of Abeta production and prevention of Abeta aggregation.

There are two approaches under investigation to reduce the production of Abeta. The first drug group under investigation is those that decrease Abeta production. These drugs, known as secretase inhibitors, target the behavior of proteins responsible for cutting the amyloid precursor protein (APP) into Abeta fragments. The second group of drugs under investigation modulates secretase, the protein responsible for splitting the APP into fragments. Although the initial trial of this type of drug was unsuccessful, there are ongoing studies targeting the modulating mechanism (Alzheimer's Association, 2007).

Abeta aggregation is of particular concern to those who treat amyloid-related diseases. Drug trials that inhibit the formation of oligomers (smaller clusters of Abeta that are still soluble) were initiated. Trials directed at blocking the aggregation of Abeta by blocking the production of oligmers were halted in 2007 because of variations in data from trial site to trial site. There is continued effort to arrest the aggregation of Abeta, with scientific investigations directed at smaller amounts of Abeta (Alzheimer's Association, 2007). There is some concern that research directed solely toward decreasing amyloid aggregation in the vessels may not be useful without restoration of the lamina of the vessel, because damaged vessels remain at risk for rupture and hemorrhage (Bugiani, 2004).

Amyloid β (Aβ) peptide immunization therapy was developed as a primary therapy to reduce amyloid levels, inhibit amyloid deposition, and clear existing plaques (Schenk et al., 1999). Although effective, several patients immunized with amyloidogenic 42-aa-long Aβ peptide (Aβ42) died during the study trial secondary to an immune response involving activated amyloid Beta and T cells (Meyer-Luehmann et al., 2010). Even though these trials were halted, they added to the body of evidence for inflammation as a clinical sequelae to CAA (Eng, Frosch, Choi, Rebeck, & Greenberg, 2004).

Summary and conclusions

Deposition of amyloid in cerebral vasculature initiates a cascade of deleterious effects including ischemia, infarction, cognitive dysfunction, and stroke. At this time, there are no specific treatments to prevent or slow the microvascular effects of CAA, although ongoing research aimed at immunosuppression, immunization, prevention of amyloid aggregation and accumulation, and other modalities may have future significance in clinical practice and prevention of AD. Recognition of persons at risk for CAA will lead to more timely diagnosis, treatment of risk factors, and prevention of the devastating consequences of CAA.

REFERENCES

Altmann-Schneider, I., Trumpet, S., de Craen, A., van Es, A., Jukema, J., et al. (2011). Cerebral microbleeds are predictive of mortality in the elderly. *Stroke, 42*, 638–644.

Alzheimer's Association (2007). Experimental Alzheimer Drugs Targeting Beta- Amyloid and the Amyloid Hypothesis. Online at: http://www.alz.org

Arima, H., Tzourio, C., Anderson, C., Woodward, M., Bousser, M., et al. (2010). Effects of perindopril-based lowering of blood pressure on intracerebral hemorrhage related to amyloid angiopathy: The PROGRESS trial. *Stroke, 41*, 394–396.

Attems, J. (2005). Sporadic cerebral amyloid angiopathy: Pathology, clinical implications, and possible pathomechanisms. *Acta Neuropathologica, 110*(4), 345–359.

Bateman, R., Munsella, L., Morris, J., Swarm, R., Yarasheski, K., & Holtzman, D. (2006). Human amyloid-β synthesis and clearance rates as measured in cerebrospinal fluid *in vivo. Nature Medicine, 12*, 856–861.

Bateman, R., Wen, G., Morris, J., & Holtzman, D. (2007). Fluctuations of CSF amyloid-β levels: Implications for a diagnostic and therapeutic biomarker. *Neurology, 69*, 1063–1065.

Bernstein, R., Gibbs, M., & Batjer, H. (2011). Clinical diagnosis and successful treatment of inflammatory cerebral amyloid angiopathy. *Neurocritical Care, 14*(3), 453–455.

Biffi, A., Halpin, A., Towfighi, A., Gilson, A., Busl, K., et al. (2010). Aspirin and recurrent intracerebral hemorrhage in cerebral amyloid angiopathy. *Neurology, 75*(8), 693–698.

Blennow, K., Hampel, H., Weiner, M., & Zetterberg, H. (2010). Cerebrospinal fluid and plasma biomarkers in Alzheimer disease. *Nature Reviews Neurology, 6*, 131–144.

Broderick, J., Connolly, S., Feldmann, E., Hanley, D., Kase, C., et al. (2007). Guidelines for the management of spontaneous intracerebral hemorrhage in adults: 2007 update: A guideline from the American Heart Association/American Stroke Association Stroke Council, High Blood Pressure Research Council, and the Quality of Care and Outcomes in Research Interdisciplinary Working Group. *Stroke, 38*(6), 2001–2023.

Bugiani, O. (2004). Aß-related cerebral angiopathy. *Neurological Sciences, 24*, S1–S2.

Chao, C., Kotsenas, A., & Broderick, D. (2006). Cerebral amyloid angiopathy: CT and MR imaging findings. *Radiographics, 26*(5), 1517–1531.

Chung, K., Anderson, N., Hutchinson, D., Synek, B., & Barber, P. (2011). Cerebral amyloid angiopathy related inflammation: Three case reports and a review. *Journal of Neurology, Neurosurgery, & Psychiatry, 82*, 20–26.

Davis. J., Xu, F., Deane, R., Romanov, G., Previti, M., et al. (2004). Early-onset and robust cerebral microvascular accumulation of amyloid β–protein in transgenic mice expressing low levels of a vasculotropic Dutch/Iowa mutant form of amyloid β-protein precursor. *Journal of Biological Chemistry, 279*, 20296–20306.

Davis, S., Broderick, J., Hennerici, M., Brun, N., Diringer, M., et al. (2006). Hematoma growth is a determinant of mortality and poor outcome after intracerebral hemorrhage. *Neurology, 66*(8), 1175–1181.

Eng, J., Frosch, M., Choi, K., Rebeck, G., & Greenberg, S. (2004). Clinical manifestations of cerebral amyloid angiopathy;related inflammation. *Annals of Neurology, 55*(2), 250–256.

Gray, F., Dubas, F., Roullet, E., & Escourolle, R. (1985). Leukoencephalopathy in diffuse hemorrhagic cerebral amyloid angiopathy. *Annals of Neurology, 18*, 54–59.

Greenberg, S. (2009). Cerebral amyloid angiopathy. In J. Carhuapoma, S. Mayer, & D. Hanley (Eds.), *Intracerebral*

Hemorrhage (pp. 41–57). New York: Cambridge University Press.

Greenberg, S. (2011). Cerebral amyloid angiopathy. Last literature review version 19.2: May.

Greenberg, S., Edip Gurol, M., Rosand, J., & Smith, E. (2004). Amyloid angiopathy-related vascular cognitive impairment. *Stroke*, *35*, 2616–2619.

Greenberg, S., Eng, J., Ning, M., Smith, E., & Rosand, J. (2004). Hemorrhage burden predicts recurrent intracerebral hemorrhage following lobar hemorrhage. *Stroke*, *35*, 1415–1420.

Greenberg S., & Levine, S. (2010). Cerebral amyloid angiography. *MedLink Neurology*. Online at: http://www.medlink.com/medlinkcontent.asp (accessed on November 15, 2010).

Greenberg, S., Schneider, A., & Pettigrew, L. (2004). Phase II study of cerebral, candidate treatment for intracerebral hemorrhage related to cerebral amyloid angiopathy. *Neurology*, *62*, A102.

Greenberg, S., Vernooij, M., Cordonnier, C., Viswanathan, A., Al-Shahi Salman, R., et al. (2009). Cerebral microbleeds: A guide to detection and interpretation. *Lancet Neurology*, *8*(2), 165–174.

Greenberg, S. & Vonsattel, J.-P. (1997). Diagnosis of cerebral amyloid angiopathy: Sensitivity and specificity of cortical biopsy. *Stroke*, *28*(7), 1418–1422.

Haglund, M., Passant, U., Sjobec, M., Ghebremedhin, E., & Englund, E. (2006). Cerebral amyloid angiopathy and cortical microinfarcts as putative substrates of vascular dementia. *International Journal of Geriatric Psychiatry*, *21*, 681–687.

Hemphill, J., Newman, J., Zhao, S., & Johnston, S. (2004). Hospital usage of early do-not-resuscitate orders and outcome after intracerebral hemorrhage. *Stroke*, *35*(5), 1130–1134.

Kinnecom, C., Lev, M., Wendell, L., Smith, E., Rosand, J., et al. (2007). Course of cerebral amyloid angiopathy-related inflammation. *Neurology*, *68*, 1411–1416.

Klein, I., Iung, B., Labreuchec, J., Hess, A., Wolff, M., et al. (2009). Cerebral microbleeds are frequent in infective endocarditis: A case-control study. *Stroke*, *40*, 3461–3465.

Kloppenborg, R., Richard, E., Sprengers, M., Troost, D., Eikelenboom, P., & Nederkoorn, P. (2010). Steroid responsive encephalopathy in cerebral amyloid angiopathy: A case report and review of evidence for immunosuppressive treatment. *Journal of Neuroinflammation, 7*, 18.

Knudsen, K., Rosand, J., Karluk, D., & Greenberg, S. (2001). Clinical diagnosis of cerebral amyloid angiopathy: Validation of the Boston criteria. *Neurology, 56*(4), 537–539.

Kumar-Singh, S. (2008). Cerebral amyloid angiopathy: Pathogenetic mechanism and link to dense amyloid plaques. *Genes, Brain and Behavior, 7*(suppl), 67–82.

Love, S., Miners, S., Palmer, J., Chalmers, K., & Kehoe, P. (2009). Insights into the pathogenesis and pathogenicity of cerebral amyloid angiopathy. *Frontiers in Bioscience, 14*, 4778–4792.

Ly, J., Donnan, G., Villemagne, Z. J., Ma, H., et al. (2010). 11C-PIB binding is increased in patients with cerebral amyloid angiopathy-related hemorrhage. *Neurology, 74*, 487–493.

Mandybur, T. (1986). Cerebral amyloid angiopathy: The vascular pathology and complications. *Journal of Neuropathology and Experimental Neurology, 45*, 79–90.

Mawuenyega, K., Sigurdson, W., Ovod, V., Munsell, L., Kasten, T., et al. (2010). Decreased clearance of CNS β-amyloid in Alzheimer's disease. *Science, 330*(6012), 1774.

McCarron, M., & Nicoll, J. (2004). Cerebral amyloid angiopathy and thrombolysis related intracerebral haemorrhage. *Lancet, 3*(8), 484–492.

Menon, R. & Kidwell, C. (2009). Neuroimaging demonstration of evolving small vessel ischemic injury in cerebral amyloid angiopathy. *Stroke, 40*(12), e675–e677.

Meyer-Luehmann, M., Mora, J., Mielke, M., Spires-Jones, T., de Calignon, A., et al. (2010). T cell mediated cerebral hemorrhages and microhemorrhages during passive $A\beta$ immunization in APPPS1 transgenic mice. *Molecular Neurodegeneration, 6*, 22.

Obici, L., Demarchi, A., de Rosa, G., Bellotti, V., Marciano, S., et al. (2005). A novel *AβPP* mutation exclusively associated with cerebral amyloid angiopathy. *Annals of Neurology, 58*, 639–644.

Petridis, A. (2008). Outcome of cerebral amyloid angiopathic brain haemorrhage. *Acta Neurochirurgica (Wein), 150*(9), 889–895.

Pettersen, J., Sathiyamoorthy, G., Gao, F., Szilagyi, G., Nadkarni, N., et al. (2008). Microbleed topography, leukoaraiosis, and cognition in probable Alzheimer disease. *Archives of Neurology, 65*(6), 790–795.

Pezzini, A., Del Zotto, E., Volonghi, I., Giossi, A., Costa, P., & Padovani, A. (2009). Cerebral amyloid angiopathy: A common cause of cerebral hemorrhage. *Current Medicinal Chemistry, 16,* 2498–2513.

Preston, S., Steart, P., Wilkinson, A., Nicoll, J., & Weller, R. (2003). Capillary and arterial cerebral amyloid angiopathy in Alzheimer's disease: Defining the perivascular route for the elimination of amyloid β from the human brain. *Neuropathology and Applied Neurobiology, 29*(2), 106–117.

Rensink, A., de Waal, R., Kremer, B., & Verbeek, M. (2003). Pathogenesis of cerebral amyloid angiopathy. *Brain Research Reviews, 43*(2), 207–223.

Rincon, F., & Mayer, S. (2008). Clinical review: Critical care management of spontaneous intracerebral hemorrhage. *Critical Care, 12*(6): 237.

Rordorf, G., & McDonald, C. (2011). Spontaneous intracerebral hemorrhage: Prognosis and treatment. Last literature review version 19.2: May 2011.

Rosand, J., Hylek, E., O'Donnell, H., & Greenberg, S. (2000). Warfarin-associated hemorrhage and cerebral amyloid angiopathy. *Neurology, 55,* 947–951.

Sacco, R., & Mayer, S. (1994). Epidemiology of intracerebral hemorrhage. In F. Armonk (Ed.), *Intracerebral Hemorrhage* (pp. 3–23). New York: Futura Publishing.

Schenk, D., Barbour, R., Dunn, W., Gordon, G., Grajeda, H., et al. (1999). Immunization with amyloid-beta attenuates Alzheimer-disease-like pathology in the PDAPP mouse. *Nature, 400*(6740), 173–177.

Schwab, P., Lidov, H., Schwartz, R., & Anderson, R. (2003). Cerebral amyloid angiopathy associated with primary angitis of the central nervous system: Report of 2 cases and review of the literature. *Arthritis Care & Research, 49*(3), 421–427.

Smith, E., & Greenberg, S. (2003). Clinical diagnosis of cerebral amyloid angiopathy: Validation of the Boston criteria. *Current Atherosclerosis Reports, 5,* 260–266.

Thanvi, B., & Robinson, T. (2006). Sporadic cerebral amyloid angiopathy-an important cause of cerebral haemorrhage in older people. *Age and Ageing, 35,* 565–571.

Towfighi, A., Greenberg, S., & Rosand, J. (2005). Treatment and prevention of primary intracerebral hemorrhage. *Seminars in Neurology*, *25*(4), 445–452.

Tsubuki, S., Takaki, Y., & Saido, T. (2003). Dutch, Flemish, Italian, and Arctic mutations of APP and resistance Abeta to physiologically relevant proteolytic degradation. *Lancet*, *361*, 1957–1958.

Verbeek, M., Kremer, B., Rikkert, M., Van Domburg, P., Skehan, M., & Greenberg, S. (2009). Cerebrospinal fluid amyloid β_{40} is decreased in cerebral amyloid angiopathy. *Annals of Neurology*, *66*(2), 245–249.

Vinters, H. (1987). Cerebral amyloid angiography: A critical review. *Stroke*, *18*, 311–324.

Viswanathan, A., Patel, P., Rahman, R., Nandigam, R., Kinnecom, C., et al. (2008). Tissue microstructural changes are independently associated with cognitive impairment in cerebral amyloid angiopathy. *Stroke*, *39*(7), 1988–1992.

Werring, D., Gregoire, S., & Cipolotti, L. (2010). Cerebral microbleeds and vascular cognitive impairment. *Journal of Neurology Science*, *299*(1–2), 131–135.

Woo, D., Sauerbeck, L., Kissela, B., Khoury, J., Szaflarski, J., et al. (2002). Genetic and environmental risk factors for intracerebral hemorrhage: Preliminary results of a population-based study. *Stroke*, *33*(5), 1190–1195.

Yamada, M. (2000). Cerebral amyloid angiopathy: An overview. *Neuropathology*, *1*, 8–22.

Vascular Malformations

7

Sheila A. Alexander

Evidence-Based Nursing Care for Stroke and Neurovascular Conditions,
First Edition. Edited by Sheila A. Alexander.
© 2013 John Wiley & Sons, Inc. Published 2013 by John Wiley & Sons, Inc.

CEREBRAL ANEURYSM
Definition and epidemiology

A cerebral aneurysm is a thin spot in a blood vessel wall of the intracranial arteries (Figure 7.1). The site of the aneurysm is weak and prone to leakage or rupture, spilling blood into the subarachnoid space and creating a life-threatening emergency. Approximately 3% of the worldwide population has an unruptured cerebral aneurysm identified on autopsy or by imaging. Up to 30% of individuals with one cerebral aneurysm have additional cerebral aneurysms. The frequency of cerebral aneurysm is fairly low, but

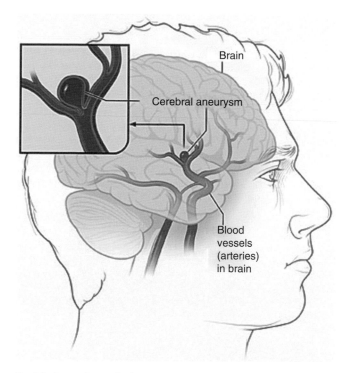

Fig. 7.1 A saccular cerebral aneurysm.
Source: http://www.nhlbi.nih.gov/health/health-topics/images/aneurysm_cerebral.jpg. Courtesy of the National Heart, Lung and Blood Institute.

the high morbidity and mortality rates associated with aneurysmal subarachnoid hemorrhage in a young population (mean age of rupture = 55 years) make this a priority for research and clinical management.

Cerebral aneurysm formation occurs at a higher frequency in individuals with certain other disorders including autosomal dominant polycystic kidney disease, fibromuscular dysplasia, Ehlers-Danlos syndrome, and Marfan syndrome. Individuals with a positive family history of subarachnoid hemorrhage or unruptured cerebral aneurysm also have a higher frequency of aneurysm development. In adults, females are more likely to harbor cerebral aneurysms (3:2) while in children, males are at higher risk. Smokers are at high risk for cerebral aneurysm and subarachnoid hemorrhage from their rupture. Individuals with two or more first-degree relatives with a cerebral aneurysm are at increased risk. Female sex and increasing age are also associated with increased risk.

Most commonly, cerebral aneurysms occur in the major cerebral blood vessels that make up the Circle of Willis (Figure 7.2). The vast majority (85%) of cerebral aneurysms develop in the anterior circulation. Most frequently, they are present in the internal carotid artery (including the posterior communicating artery), followed by the middle cerebral artery, anterior cerebral artery, and vertebral and basilar arteries (Vlak, Algra, Brandenburg, & Rinkel, 2011). Aneurysms greater than 5 mm in size are at increased risk for rupture and subarachnoid hemorrhage. Aneurysms in the posterior circulation (posterior inferior cerebellar arteries, vertebral arteries, and basilar artery) are at higher risk for rupture at a smaller size (see Figure 7.2). Additionally, higher rates of subarachnoid hemorrhage without an increase frequency of intracranial aneurysms have been found in Japanese and Finnish populations (Vlak et al., 2011).

Pathophysiology

The pathologic mechanism of aneurysm development is not known. It is likely a complex process involving environmental, genetic, and epigenetic exposures. The unique features of the cerebral blood vessels may contribute to the development of aneurysms. The median muscularis layer is absent at bifurcations of cerebral

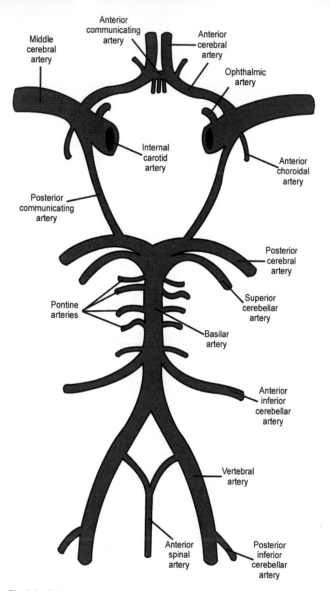

Fig. 7.2 Circle of Willis. Adapted from Lewis, W. H. (Ed.). (1918). Anatomy of the human body. Philadelphia, PA: Lea & Febiger. Adapted from Lewis, W. H (Ed.). (1918). Anatomy of the human body. Philadelphia, PA: Lea & Febiger. Available from Wikimedia Commons at http://en.wikipedia.org/wiki/File:Circle_of_Willis_en.svg.

vessels, a common place for aneurysm development. The cerebral vasculature contains fragile or absence of external elastic lamina, which provides support and strength to arteries in other areas of the body. Defective collagen and elastin have been identified at varying levels in cerebral arteries with greatest defects in ruptured aneurysms, followed by unruptured aneurysms and then cerebral arteries without aneurysms. Improper collagen and elastin are hypothesized to create weaker blood vessel walls and promote aneurysm formation. Additional work suggests that arterial repair mechanisms are insufficient in some individuals, resulting in the formation of aneurysms at sites where there is a high level of shear stress and vascular damage without proper repair. Currently there is no clear consensus, and it is likely that multiple cellular-level events occur leading to aneurysm formation. Atherosclerosis is also a potential cause of aneurysms, and in particular fusiform aneurysms. Infection, trauma, and drugs may also lead to aneurysm formation.

In many individuals the cerebral aneurysm exists without causing any problems and will likely go undiagnosed. There are several scenarios that result in cerebral aneurysm identification. The most common, and life-threatening, is subarachnoid hemorrhage where the aneurysm ruptures leading to a hemorrhagic stroke. See Chapter 5 for care of the patient recovering from subarachnoid hemorrhage. Some aneurysms present as pain behind the eye, cranial nerve paralysis, or headache or neck pain due to leakage of blood from the aneurysm without full rupture. Often called a "sentinel bleed" due to the presence of a small subarachnoid blood, the aneurysm identified in this manner should be treated promptly to prevent an actual rupture and larger subarachnoid hemorrhage resulting in a poor outcome. Some aneurysms present due to third nerve palsy, visual loss (ophthalmic artery aneurysm), or brainstem compression (due to a giant aneurysm). These are emergent conditions with higher rupture risk that require immediate aneurysm securement. Cerebral aneurysms may also present with symptoms of fatigue, loss of balance, perceptual disturbances, speech problems, and double vision. A small portion of aneurysms are identified serendipitously when the patient has radiographic testing for another cause (e.g., a computed tomography (CT) scan after a car accident with suspicion of head injury).

Monitoring and rupture prevention

All cerebral aneurysms that rupture should receive emergency care (see Chapter 5). Most aneurysms are not life threatening. The risk of rupture of a cerebral aneurysm has been estimated at 0.5–2% per year, but certain characteristics including increased aneurysm size and location can increase this risk considerably (Juvela, Porras, & Heiskanen, 1993; Juvela, Poussa, & Porras, 2001; Winn, Jane Sr., Taylor, Kaiser, & Britz, 2002; Wiebers et al., 2003). Larger aneurysms and those in the posterior circulation are more likely to rupture (Juvela, Porras, & Heiskanen, 1993). Additionally, aneurysms in patients who have previously had a subarachnoid hemorrhage are more likely to rupture. Once the aneurysm has been identified, treatment decisions are made based on size, location (and often growth rate) of the aneurysms, patient age, medical history, previous subarachnoid hemorrhage, and cigarette smoking status (Juvela, Porras, & Poussa, 2000; Juvella, 2003; Wiebers et al., 2003).

The care of the patient with a symptomatic aneurysm should be focused on relieving the symptoms and decreasing the risk of rupture. If a patient has pain or headaches, non-steroidal anti-inflammatory drugs (NSAIDs) have been found to be helpful in this population. In general, symptomatic unruptured aneurysms should be secured to prevent rupture and decrease symptoms.

Certainly any patient with an unruptured cerebral aneurysm should avoid increases in blood pressure. Anti-hypertensive medications should be utilized to maintain a normal blood pressure, below 120/80 mmHg. Additional lifestyle modifications including regular exercise and a low-fat, low-sodium diet may be adequate to maintain blood pressure at a low risk level. Cigarette smoking is a risk factor for aneurysmal subarachnoid hemorrhage; individuals with unruptured cerebral aneurysms should stop smoking.

Digital subtraction angiography (DSA) is the gold standard for identification and classification of cerebral aneurysms. A cerebral aneurysm will show as a contrast-filled outpouching on the vessel. Due to the invasive nature of DSA, other neuroimaging methods are often used to locate size and position, and to monitor growth of cerebral aneurysm. Standard CT scanning without contrast may identify large aneurysms (>10 mm) or calcified aneurysms; however, this is not ideal as most unruptured aneurysms are smaller and would not be detected with this technology. CT scan with contrast will show the aneurysm as a well-defined isodense or hyperdense figure in the subarachnoid space. A partially thrombosed aneurysm may appear differently, as contrast will collect around the thrombosed area, outlining the internal lumen and edges of the aneurysm. CT angiographic (CTA) techniques can be used to provide angiographic-like images of unruptured aneurysms. CTA utilizes rapid dye infusion and dynamic CT scanning to generate images of excellent quality. Aneurysm location, size (>3 mm), and relationship to the parent vessel can be determined. CTA technology provides a three-dimensional image showing vasculature, including the aneurysm, in the context of brain tissue, bone, and fluid. Magnetic resonance imaging (MRI) can also be used to identify and monitor unruptured cerebral aneurysms. Aneurysms appear as either hyperintense or hypointense signals depending on flow characteristics and specific MRI technology used. On a T1-T2 weighted imaging, aneurysms appear as a well-defined mass, although heterogeneity may be present for aneurysms with turbulent flow. Thrombosed aneurysms often appear as hyperintense within the lumen and variable intensities in surrounding areas. Magnetic resonance angiography (MRA) creates more detailed images of the intracranial space. MRA can identify the size and location of the aneurysm, as well as its relationship to the parent vessel and surrounding tissue, in a three-dimensional image.

Upon identification of an unruptured aneurysm, care is variable depending on the aneurysm's size and location, and other clinical characteristics of the individual patient.

Small aneurysms (<3 mm)
Smaller, unruptured aneurysms smaller than 3 mm warrant serial CTA or MRA scanning to monitor for increase growth. There is no standard timeframe for such evaluation, but it has been recommended that annual screening may be adequate to monitor for growth in aneurysms that are of this size.

Medium aneurysms (3–7 mm)
For aneurysms 3–7 mm in size in individuals over 65 years old, risk should be considered. If there is no previous history of cerebral aneurysm rupture, no family history of subarachnoid hemorrhage,

and no diagnosis of autosomal dominant polycystic kidney disease, monitoring is warranted. Individuals over 65 years old with aneurysms 3–7 mm in size and a previous subarachnoid hemorrhage from an aneurysm, autosomal dominant polycystic kidney disease, and family history of subarachnoid hemorrhage *or* without these risk factors but with significant anxiety related to having an untreated, unruptured aneurysm, aneurysm securement should be considered.

Individuals with aneurysms 3–7 mm in size who are less than 65 years old likely should be treated. If the aneurysm is in a high risk location or a difficult to secure surgically, the decision to treat must be weighed based on additional factors. Location of the aneurysm, and associated risk, should be considered. Aneurysms not in high-risk locations, in individuals who are not at increased risk due to previous personal or family history, may be monitored with CTA or MRA every 12 months. For aneurysms in a high-risk location and/or individuals at increased risk due to personal or family history, decision to treat with coil embolization or surgical clipping aneurysms in a difficult location for surgical securement may be better treated with coil embolization. Coil embolization of these aneurysms may be ideal for settings with experienced personnel (typically a neuro-radiologist, interventional radiologist, or neurosurgeon/neurologist with experience and skill in embolization). Availability of a neurosurgeon with expertise and experience is necessary for surgical securement and in particularly if the aneurysm is in a difficult surgical location. These patients should be monitored with CTA or MRA every 12 months if the aneurysm is not secured.

Large aneurysms (> 7 mm)
Aneurysms larger than 7 mm are at risk for rupture, and decision making should lead to treatment either with surgical clipping or endovascular coiling.

Treatment of individuals age 70 or older with aneurysms larger than 7 mm but smaller than 25 mm in size and without symptoms must be weighed in the context of general health, surgical/treatment risk, and life expectancy. If the individual is in poor general health, is at high risk of morbidity related to anesthesia required, and/or has a terminal illness, monitoring with CTA or MRA versus no treatment of the aneurysm should be considered.

Individuals younger than 70 years, with aneurysms larger than 7 mm but less than 25 mm in size and without symptoms should be treated. If the aneurysm lies within a surgically difficult location and a neurosurgeon with significant expertise and experience in surgical securement is available, surgery or coil embolization should be considered. If there is not a neurosurgeon with significant expertise and experience available coil embolization is the preferred method of treatment. If the aneurysm is not within a surgically difficult location, surgery versus coil embolization treatment options should still be considered.

Aneurysm size

Small aneurysms (<7 mm) should be monitored periodically for increase in size. Typically CT scan or MRI is performed every 3–12 months. The rate of aneurysm growth may be helpful in predicting which aneurysms will go on to rupture, and provide clues as to when intervention is necessary to ablate the aneurysm to prevent hemorrhage. Some aneurysms do not appear to grow, and it is impossible to predict when an aneurysm will begin to grow or when it might rupture. Current evidence suggests that a symptomatic, unruptured cerebral aneurysm in an otherwise healthy individual should be secured via surgical or endovascular therapies(Juvela, Porras, & Poussa, 2000; Wiebers et al., 2003). Larger aneurysms (>7 mm) require more frequent neurologic monitoring and should be secured in individuals of all ages regardless of symptom presentation (Juvela, Porras, & Poussa, 2000).

Aneurysm location

Cerebral aneurysms in select locations are at increased risk of rupture. Aneurysms within the posterior circulation (posterior inferior cerebellar, vertebral, or basilar arteries) or the posterior communicating arteries are at high risk for rupture. Aneurysms within the posterior circulation, paraclinoid aneurysms (ophthalmic, super hypophyseal), and aneurysms larger than 12 mm in size are considered to be difficult to secure surgically.

Aneurysm securement methods
Coil embolization

The development of coil embolization in 1991 has significantly improved outcome for patients who are poor surgical risks or have aneurysms that are not able to be secured with typical surgical techniques. While this is a relatively new procedure, evidence supports it is as safe and effective for aneurysm securement, and it is associated with similar outcomes for patients undergoing surgical aneurysm securement. Recent evidence has shown that coil embolization of aneurysms in patients in good health is associated with improved outcomes, although this work was done in patients who suffered aneurysmal subarachnoid hemorrhage (Van der Schaaf et al., 2009). Whether this relates to a decreased risk of infection, reduction of anesthesia required for embolization, or some other factor is unclear. Coil embolization is considered in many circumstances including: (1) presence of fusiform or berry aneurysms with a wide neck that are difficult to treat with a surgical clip; (2) posterior circulation aneurysms that are more difficult to treat surgically as more brain must be displaced to reach the aneurysm; and (3) in patients who are not likely to tolerate surgery.

Coil embolization is performed by a neurosurgeon or an interventional neuro-radiologist who has had additional training in this procedure. An angiographic catheter is threaded through femoral artery into the internal carotid artery and up into the cranial vault during typical angiography. Radio-opaque dye is injected into the vessels and fills distal vessels, thereby identifying vascular abnormalities that fill with dye. A special catheter is threaded through the vessels and into the aneurysm. A charge of electricity travels through the catheter and releases the coil into the aneurysm. This procedure must be performed repeatedly until the aneurysm is filled with coils. Finally, an additional electric charge is transmitted through the catheter to initiate blood coagulation. Once the aneurysm is filled with coils, blood no longer flows through the aneurysm and it is no longer at risk of rupture. Coil embolization assumes the same risks as traditional cerebral angiography including hemorrhage due to puncture of a vessel, hematoma formation at the catheterization site, anesthesia-related complications, and infection, although less anesthesia is used and infection risk is lower as compared to surgical management. Additional risk is incurred as, rarely, coils may detach and be sent to areas outside the aneurysm.

Patients recovering from coil embolization do not routinely require care in an intensive care unit setting. Frequent neurologic assessment should be performed (every 1–2 hours) to monitor for complications and untoward anesthesia effects. If the angiographic catheter has been left in the patient, it should be connected to a pressure monitor with alarm settings calibrated to identify blood pressure greater than the upper limit identified above, but also to identify a significant drop in blood pressure that could impair cerebral perfusion and catheter disconnect/dislodgement. Angiographic catheters are large and can lead to significant bleeding if dislodged. A properly placed catheter can leak and lead to hematoma formation. Catheter placement site should be covered with an occlusive dressing and the insertion site should be monitored periodically (every 5–15 minutes for the first 1–2 hours, then every 1–2 hours until removal) for leakage or hematoma. If blood is to be drawn from this line, sterile blood draw procedures should be used and care should be taken to prevent catheter dislodgement. If the catheter has been removed, as in most cases, the catheter site should be monitored every 5–15 minutes for 1–2 hours, then every 1–2 hours for at least 8 hours, then every 2–4 hours for 24 hours.

Surgical securement

Despite advancements in angiographic procedures, surgical clipping remains the most prominent form of aneurysm securement. During this procedure, the surgeon must drill through bone, remove a section of it, and displace brain tissue to visualize the aneurysm. Once the aneurysm is visible, surgical clips are placed at the neck of the aneurysm to prevent blood from flowing into the aneurysm and the dome of the aneurysm is nicked to assure no blood enters the aneurysm. Historically, aneurysms were wrapped with gauze (to promote scar tissue formation around the aneurysm) or ligated for securement. While these procedures are rarely performed since the development of the surgical clip, there are times when they are preferable, providing a less dangerous procedure to the patient or more effective securement of the aneurysm. Aneurysms in the anterior circulation and berry-type aneurysms are more amenable to surgical clipping. Patients having surgical securement of cerebral aneurysms are still at risk for complications commonly associated with anesthesia and surgery including infection.

Post-operative care

Patients recovering from brain surgery for aneurysm securement do not necessarily require an intensive care unit setting. Patients in good general health having unruptured aneurysm securement via surgical clipping can be extubated in the post-anesthesia care unit and transferred to a general surgical unit for monitoring up to 24 hours and discharged to home. In the first 24 hours, frequent neurologic assessment should be performed (every 1–2 hours) to monitor for complications and untoward anesthesia effects.

ARTERIOVENOUS MALFORMATION
Definition and epidemiology

An arteriovenous malformation (AVM) is a large group of arteries and veins that are joined without a capillary bed. AVMs vary in size and presentation. Approximately 0.89 to 1.34 per 100,000 people are thought to have cerebral AVMs worldwide, although a recent Scottish study reported an estimated prevalence of 18/100,000. There has not been consistent reporting of AVM frequency in other populations worldwide and it appears there is significant variability. AVMs present equally in males and females and in people of all racial and ethnic backgrounds equally and usually before the third decade of life. AVMs are at higher risk for hemorrhage due to the weak vessel walls.

Only about 12% of individuals with an AVM will have symptoms. Nearly 50% of symptomatic AVMs present as intracerebral hemorrhage (ICH). Children are seven times more likely to present with ICH as compared to seizures. Seizures are the second most common presentation followed by headaches and focal neurologic symptoms. Patients with known AVMs have a hemorrhage rate of 2–18%. The variability in this rate is due to the minimal research systematically examining hemorrhage rates. Children and adolescents, and some adults, with AVMs may exhibit learning disorders or behavioral disorders. Some patients may have a bruit. Pregnant women who harbor AVMs may experience symptoms or ICH for the first time due to the increased blood volume and blood pressure associated with pregnancy.

Pathophysiology

It is not clear what causes the development of an AVM. They are thought to be congenital or present from birth, although the mechanisms of how an AVM develops is not known. The increased velocity of the blood coming into the AVM from the arterial flow through the venous side of the abnormality causes the veins to dilate and weaken. The weak venous walls are likely to rupture, dumping blood into the parenchyma and in some instanced the ventricles and subarachnoid space. The blood load from a bleeding AVM is very large, causing intracranial pressure problems, herniation, and death in approximately 10% of cases. Subsequent ICH is associated with increasing mortality rates.

Smaller AVMs, those with limited or impaired drainage systems, and AVMs that have previously ruptured are at increased risk for hemorrhage. An AVM in a pregnant woman is also at increased risk for hemorrhage. Many AVMs, particularly those that are large, cause symptoms for other reasons. The large size of a growing AVM can put pressure on nearby structures and cause increased ICP. Because they are extremely vascular, they also command a greater proportion of the blood and may divert blood away from healthy brain tissue, leading to symptoms including seizures. The specific symptoms of an AVM depend on the location as well.

Management

The management of the patient with an AVM is variable depending on the size of the AVM, location, presence/absence of symptoms, and risk of rupture. For some small AVMs, monitoring is adequate to ensure there is no growth or additional blood flow burden. If the patient becomes symptomatic or the AVM increases in size, there are a few treatment options available.

Diagnosis and monitoring

Diagnosis of AVM requires radiographic imaging. CT scan technology is an ideal screening tool for patients presenting with neurologic symptoms suggestive of an AVM. CT scan can demonstrate the location and size of the lesion, any acute hemorrhage, and presence of hydrocephalus. Unruptured AVMs present as an irregular hyperdensity, often with calcification. MRI scanning can provide additional information showing more detailed architecture of the AVM. MRI shows the AVM, but also its nidus, feeding arteries, draining veins, and the relationship to nearby brain structures. On T1-T2 weighted images, an AVM appears as a porous structure with feeding arterial and venous vessels. If the AVM has ruptured, blood clots may obscure the AVM on an MRI.

Once an AVM has been identified, cerebral angiography must be performed to inform treatment decisions. Cerebral angiography shows the AVM, its nidus, arterial feeders and venous drainage system, the relationship to other brain structures, and associated cerebral aneurysms. Cerebral angiography should be performed as part of the preoperative evaluation, because AVMs change over time and the local geography may be different than it was at initial diagnosis.

The specific treatment selected must consider many factors. Surgical resection can generally be done in a single treatment, and is therefore preferred over other methods that require multiple treatments over longer periods of time. Cerebellar, brainstem, basal ganglia, and thalamic AVMs are at high risk of hemorrhage, in addition to high mortality in the face of hemorrhage, so prompt repair is required. They are also in locations that make surgery difficult, so an experienced neurosurgeon is needed. The venous drainage system should also be considered. AVMs with a single draining vein, stenosis, or kinking of the venous drainage system are at high risk of hemorrhage. Presence of aneurysms in addition to an AVM is an additional risk factor for hemorrhage. Patient's age must also be considered. Risk of hemorrhage over a lifetime is higher in younger patients, and children respond better to neurologic injury, so pediatric patients with an AVM should be a high priority for surgical treatment. Poor baseline health and increased patient's age may impact surgical risk such that the risk of surgery becomes greater than the risk of hemorrhage. Patient lifestyle and occupation also must be considered. Surgical AVM resection often destroys nearby brain tissue. If a surgical procedure will destroy tissue vital to the patient's lifestyle and occupation, alternative treatments may be preferred. The location or size of the AVM may not be conducive to surgical treatment.

Surgical treatments

AVMs are frequently resected surgically. Preoperative care of the patient requiring surgical resection of the AVM calls for pre-anesthesia care (NPO after midnight, history and physical), but there are no AVM-specific requirements. Cerebral angiography should occur as part of the preoperative work up to facilitate optimal surgical approach.

The surgical procedure requires the neurosurgeon reduce the AVM by vessel resection. AVM resection begins with a removal of a portion of the skull and, unless the AVM is on the surface of the brain, displacement of brain tissue to reach the AVM. The surgeon then resects the AVM by individual vessels. This is a lengthy procedure with an 8% mortality rate. Simple resection is most frequently performed if the AVM is small and superficial.

Patients recovering from brain surgery for AVM resection do not necessarily require an intensive care unit setting. Patients in good general health having AVM resection can be extubated in the post-anesthesia care unit and transferred to a general surgical unit for monitoring up to 24 hours and discharged to home. In the first 24 hours, frequent neurologic assessment should be performed (every 1–2 hours) to monitor for complications and untoward anesthesia effects. Long-term follow-up should include repeat CTA, MRA, or cerebral angiography to ensure successful resection has occurred and no regrowth had developed.

Embolization

Embolization of an AVM is becoming more frequent. Pre-procedural care requires standard pre-anesthesia care (NPO after midnight, history and physical), but there are no AVM-specific requirements.

Embolization is performed by a neurosurgeon or an interventional neuro-radiologist who has had additional training in this procedure. An angiographic catheter is threaded through femoral artery into one or more feeding arteries. An embolizing agent is then injected into the AVM. Embolizing agents include fast-drying, biologically inert glues, fibered titanium coils, and tiny balloons. Embolization does not always permanently obliterate the AVM. Embolization is frequently used in combination with surgery or radiosurgery. Embolization shrinks the AVM and reduces blood flow through it, making surgical techniques safer. Embolization assumes the same risks as traditional cerebral angiography, including hemorrhage due to puncture of a vessel, hematoma formation at the catheterization site, anesthesia-related complications, and infection. Risk is lower due to a decreased need for anesthesia and a lower infection risk.

Patients recovering from coil embolization do not routinely require care in an intensive care unit setting. Frequent neurologic assessment should be performed (every 1–2 hours) to monitor for complications and untoward anesthesia effects. If the angiographic catheter has been left in the patient, it should be connected to a pressure monitor with alarm settings calibrated to identify blood pressure greater than the upper limit identified above, but also to identify a significant drop in blood pressure that could impair cerebral perfusion and catheter disconnect/dislodgement. Angiographic catheters are large and can lead to significant bleeding if dislodged. A properly placed catheter can leak and lead to hematoma formation. Catheter placement site should be covered with an occlusive dressing and the insertion site should be monitored periodically (every 5–15 minutes for the first 1–2 hours, then every 1–2 hours until removal) for leakage or hematoma. If blood is to be drawn from this line, sterile blood draw procedures should be used and care should be taken to prevent catheter dislodgement. If the catheter has been removed, as in most cases, the catheter site should be monitored every 5–15 minutes for 1–2 hours, then every 1–2 hours for at least 8 hours, then every 2–4 hours for 24 hours.

Radiosurgery

Radiosurgery is a procedure frequently used for large and deep AVMs. Radiosurgery is performed by a neurosurgeon or interventional neuro-radiologist. A highly focused beam of radiation is directed at the AVM, damaging the walls of the blood vessels within the AVM. Radiosurgery ablation of an AVM requires multiple doses provided over a period of several months. Repeated treatments cause a gradual breakdown of the vessels and resolution of the AVM.

CEREBRAL CAVERNOUS MALFORMATION
Definition and epidemiology

A cerebral cavernous malformation (CCM) is a collection of capillaries, similar to an AVM but made up of veins without arterial support, that can develop anywhere within the central nervous system. CCMs are also called cavernous angiomas or cavernomas. CCMs are present in about 1 of every 200 people. They develop in males and females equally and in people of all races and ages. CCMs most often present between the ages of 10 years and 40 years. While a person may have only one CCM, it is common to have multiple CCMs. Most CCMs occur in the intracranial vault, brain, or brainstem, with 5–10% occurring in the spinal cord (Deutsch, Jallo, Faktorovich, & Epstein, 2000).

Many CCMs are asymptomatic for the lifespan of the individual. Approximately 50–75% of CCMs will present with symptoms, although research identifying CCM on autopsy indicate a much higher number of asymptomatic CCM. Common symptoms of a CCM are seizures. Other symptoms include headaches, visual changes, hearing changes, and paralysis. About 32% of CCMs bleed into the cranial vault, brain stem, or spinal cord (Denier et al., 2004). Fatality rates from a CCM are related to its risk of hemorrhage and surgical intervention. A presentation of CCM with fatal hemorrhage is rare. Repeated small hemorrhagic events frequently occur before a large, life-threatening hemorrhage.

Pathophysiology

CCMs create caverns, or open spaces, within the capillary. These caverns are filled with blood. The blood within the caverns may also form a thrombus, blocking blood flow through the area. The walls of the vessels of the CCM, and the caverns in particular, are lined with a single layer of epithelium and lack a muscle layer. This makes the walls very thin and prone to bleeding. CCMs frequently have small hemorrhages or leaking of blood from the lesion that may or may not result in symptoms. Larger hemorrhages do occur and can be life threatening depending on the size and location. Bleeding into the brainstem region is particularly life threatening. Blood, and products produced during its breakdown, can compress nearby tissue, leading to symptoms. Hemosiderin is one such by-product that is present in the tissue around a CCM. Evidence suggests there is a loss of blood brain barrier within this region, promoting vascular instability.

There is an autosomal dominant heritability associated with approximately 20% of CCM cases. Research has suggested that several genetic mutations may be associated with CCM development, which informs our understanding of the pathways involved in their development, specifically, mutations that result in loss of function of the CCM1 (Krit), CCM2 (Osmosensing scaffold for MEKK3-OSM, Malcavernin, or MGC4607) and CCM3 (or PCD10) gene products. The mutated gene products result in endothelial cell junction integrity, RhoA hyperactivation, and resultant endothelial cell – and ultimately vascular – instability.

Signs and symptoms of a CCM are due to one of a few processes. Irritation of the surrounding tissue, produced by hemorrhage and/or inflammation, produces seizure activity. A large CCM may compress surrounding tissues, leading to seizures or focal neurologic deficit.

Management

Diagnosis of a CCM requires a neurologic examination when symptoms present, along with a complete medical and family history. A familial history of two or more family members with CCM is strongly suggestive of the familial form of CCM. The CCM shows clearly on MRI scanning, particularly when brain gradient echo (GRE) or susceptibility-weighted imaging (SWI) are employed. A CCM appears as a multi-globular lesion with a complex core of mixed signal intensities suggesting hemorrhage of varying age. A small portion of CCMs are identified before they express symptoms. It is estimated that these serendipitously discovered lesions have a hemorrhage rate of less than 1% per year. Serendipitously identified CCMs and those presenting with mild symptoms may be monitored with annual MRI scanning to monitor for changes within the lesion. Serial monitoring is used to identify new lesions, or new or growing hemorrhage within or near the lesion. There is currently no method to determine if or when a CCM will hemorrhage or begin to exhibit symptoms.

While there is not empirical evidence supporting these practices, most clinicians agree that the following practices should be employed in patients with asymptomatic CCM. Maintaining blood pressure in the low-normal range, avoiding blood-thinning agents such as aspirin, heparin, or sodium warfarin, and avoiding NSAIDS and activities where the patient is subject to strong gravitational force (such as a roller coaster or centrifugal force rides) develop healthy stress management techniques. Acetaminophen is an acceptable pain relief agent for patients with CCM.

Anti-epileptic medications

Seizure management in a symptomatic patient is warranted. Surgical resection of the CCM may be warranted for individuals with an accessible CCM (see Surgical Intervention section). There is no specific anti-epileptic/anti-convulsant recommended specifically for patients with CCM. Rather, a drug that stops seizure activity with minimal side effects and considering the patients baseline medical status should be utilized.

Surgical intervention

Surgical intervention for CCM is warranted for patients who have recurrent hemorrhage, progressive or severe symptoms, or seizures not responsive to therapy. Patient's age and medical history, lesion size and complexity, as well as location are considered by the surgeon/surgical team when making the decision about surgical intervention. Brainstem lesions are generally only resected when they produce symptoms and lie against a pial or ependymal surface. Surgical treatment is very effective in excising the lesion and alleviating symptoms, but only if the entire lesion is removed. Incomplete lesion removal is associated with regrowth of the lesion, recurrence of hemorrhage, and symptoms.

Preoperative care of the patient requiring surgical resection of CCM calls for standard pre-anesthesia care including a full history and physical. The patient should be kept NPO after midnight or for several hours before surgery.

The surgical procedure frequently utilizes a stereotactic navigation system to localize the site and orientation of the lesion. A small craniotomy site is created and minimal (if any) tissue is displaced. CCMs frequently reside near the surface of the cortex and close to a fissure or sulcus, so little brain tissue must be displaced. Once the CCM is localized, it is partially resected and cauterized to promote coagulation. Repeat resection and cauterization are performed until the entire lesion is removed. Surgical resection of supratentorial lesions has an extremely low mortality rate and excellent morbidity rate, with few patients experiencing permanent deficit. Surgical resection of brainstem CCMs by an experienced surgeon is associated with a low mortality rate (4%) and 12% permanent deficit rate (Zabramski & Spetzler, 2003).

Surgical intervention for CCM requires a short stay in the hospital. Admission to an intensive care unit setting should be made on a case-by-case basis and generally is only required for patients with significant medical histories or complications. Patients in good general health can be extubated in the post-anesthesia care unit and transferred to a general surgical unit for monitoring for 48–72 hours. Monitoring should include frequent vital signs, neurologic assessment, and physical examination (every 1–2 hours) to monitor for complications and anesthesia effects. Patients exhibiting no adverse effects may have less frequent monitoring. Most patients recover without incident and are able to be discharged to home in 2–3 days, returning to work and normal activity in 2–3 weeks. Physical therapy is helpful in regaining function for patients who have focal neurologic deficits.

Ongoing research

Statins are HMG-CoA reductase inhibitors. HMG-CoA reductase inihibits cholesterol formation and the formation of gerranyl-geranyl-diphosphate, a lipid required for proper functioning of RhoA. Current research is exploring the efficacy of statin use in stabilizing and perhaps reversing a CCM.

Evidence is growing for the potential use of propranolol, a beta-adrenergic receptor blocker, to treat CCMs.

Fadusil, a Rho kinase inhibitor, has also shown promise in preventing lesion development in animal models (McDonald et al., 2012).

Stereotactic radiosurgery is another method currently under investigation for treating CCMs. This method requires a brief radiation treatment focused on the CCM, similar to what is required for an arterial venous malformation. Long-term monitoring of these patients to determine potential long-term effects of radiation treatment and permanent ablation of the lesion is ongoing.

REFERENCES

Denier, C., Labauge, P., Brunereau, L., et al. (2004). Clinical features of cerebral cavernous malformations patients with KRIT1 mutations. *Annals of Neurology, 55*(2), 213–220.

Deutsch, H., Jallo, G. I., Faktorovich, A., & Epstein, F. (2000). Spinal intramedullary cavernoma: Clinical presentation and surgical outcome. *Journal of Neurosurgery, 93*(1 Suppl), 65–70.

Juvela, S. (2003). Prehemorrhage risk factors for fatal intracranial aneurysm rupture. *Stroke, 34*(8), 1852–1857.

Juvela, S., Porras, M., & Heiskanen, O. (1993). Natural history of unruptured intracranial aneurysms: A long-term follow-up study. *Journal of Neurosurgery, 79*(2), 174–182.

Juvela, S., Porras, M., & Poussa, K. (2000). Natural history of unruptured intracranial aneurysms: Probability and risk factors for aneurysm rupture. *Neurosurgical Focus, 8*(5), Preview 1.

Juvela, S., Poussa, K., & Porras, M. (2001). Factors affecting formation and growth of intracranial aneurysms: A long-term follow-up study. *Stroke, 32*(2), 485–491.

McDonald, D. A., Shi, C., Shenkar, R., et al. (2012). Fasudil decreases lesion burden in a murine model of crebral cavernous malformation disease. *Stroke, 43*, 571–574.

Van der Schaaf, I., Algra, A., Wermer, M., Molyneux, A., Clarke, M. J. (2009). Endovascular coiling versus neurosurgical clipping for patients with aneurysmal subarachnoid haemorrhage. *The Cochrane Library.* DOI: 10.1002/14651858.CD003085.pub2.

Vlak, M. H., Algra, A., Brandenburg, R., & Rinkel, G. J. (2011). Prevalence of unruptured intracranial aneurysms, with emphasis on sex, age, comorbidity, country, and time period: A systematic review and meta-analysis. *Lancet Neurology, 10*(7), 626–636.

Wiebers, D. O., Whisnant, J. P., Huston III, J., et al. (2003). Unruptured intracranial aneurysms: Natural history, clinical outcome, and risks of surgical and endovascular treatment. *Lancet, 362*(9378), 103–110.

Winn, H. R., Jane Sr., J. A., Taylor, J., Kaiser, D., & Britz, G. W. (2002). Prevalence of asymptomatic incidental aneurysms: Review of 4568 arteriograms. *Journal of Neurosurgery, 96*(1), 43–49.

Zabramski, J. M., & Spetzler, R. F. (2003). Cavernous malformations. In A. Daroff (Ed.), *Encyclopedia of the Neurological Sciences* (pp. 532–538). New York: Academic Press.

Cerebral Autosomal Dominant Arteriopathy with Subcortical Infarcts and Leukoencephalopathy (CADASIL)

8

Sheila A. Alexander

Evidence-Based Nursing Care for Stroke and Neurovascular Conditions,
First Edition. Edited by Sheila A. Alexander.
© 2013 John Wiley & Sons, Inc. Published 2013 by John Wiley & Sons, Inc.

Cerebral Autosomal Dominant Arteriopathy with Subcortical Infarcts and Leukoencephalopathy (CADASIL) is an inherited disorder hallmarked by degeneration of the smooth muscle cells of the cerebral blood vessels resulting in white matter destruction/degeneration, migraines, mood disorders, and early-age stroke, ultimately progressing to early-age dementia. Additional symptoms of this disease are variable and include seizures, cognitive deterioration, depression, and personality/behavioral changes. Most individuals suffering CADASIL present with symptoms in their early thirties but some present later in life. Symptoms are progressive, with most patients suffering multiple strokes, dementia, and often motor deficits (as a result of stroke to the primary motor strip or diencephalon structures) by age 65.

PATHOPHYSIOLOGY

Like all autosomal dominant disorders, CADASIL requires an individual inherit only one copy of the variant (less common) allele of the gene. The gene responsible for CADASIL is "Notch 3," a gene on chromosome 19, encoding neurogenic locus notch homolog protein 3. Neurogenic locus notch homolog protein 3 is a protein expressed as a surface receptor by only smooth muscle cells of the arterial vasculature. It is highly involved in blood vessel development and maintenance. Neurogenic locus notch homolog protein 3 expression and accumulation in the cytoplasm of muscle cells lining the cerebral vasculature leads to hypertrophy and dysfunction of these cells.

During normal functioning, cells produce proteins to carry out required functions of that cell type via transcription and translation. Transcription and translation of the Notch 3 gene result in production of neurogenic locus notch homolog protein 3. The variant form of the Notch 3 gene produces a functionally different neurogenic locus notch homolog protein 3. The variant protein is not easily broken up and eliminated from the cell. Buildup of this protein in the cytoplasm, near the cell membrane, increases the size of the individual cell. As multiple smooth muscle cells of the vasculature increase in size and the protein builds up, the internal lumen of the blood vessels narrows and predisposes to alterations in blood flow. Lacunar strokes are quite common, with hemispheric strokes occurring in a minority of the population. Repeated small strokes that may not be evidenced by clinical symptoms contribute to cell loss with resultant cognitive decline and dementia seen in later stages of the disease.

SYMPTOMS

In about one-third of individuals with CADASIL, migraine is the presenting symptom (Desmond et al., 1999; Vahedi et al., 2004). Cognitive deficits, and particularly impairment of executive functioning, are a common presenting symptom in many patients (Dichgans et al., 1998; Buffon et al., 2006). Additional cognitive deficits develop over time as the disease progresses. Mood and psychiatric disorders are the frequently presenting symptoms of patients with CADASIL (Vahedi et al., 2004). Seizures are the presenting symptom in a minority of CADASIL patients (Desmond, Tatemichi, Paik, & Stern, 1993).

Symptoms of CADASIL often begin with migraine headaches at age 20–40. They occur in up to 40% of individuals with CADASIL. Neuropsychiatric symptoms are present throughout the disease process. Mood disorders are diagnosed in 10–20% of these patients. Major depression is the most common mood disorder seen in individuals with CADASIL, presenting in about 10% of the population at some point during their lives. Few individuals with CADASIL develop bipolar disorder and major depressive episode(s) alternating with manic episode(s). Agoraphobia, alcohol abuse, and psychoses have been reported (Chabriat et al., 1995; Verin et al., 1995; Dichgans et al., 1998). A decrease in cognitive functioning typically occurs after age 50, although recent evidence suggests a decline in memory function may present as early as age 35. Other cognitive domains are lost in disease progression, such that language skills, instrumental functioning and visuospatial impairment develop. While cognitive alterations may be caused by an ischemic event, for many CADASIL patients these changes occur before a diagnosis of stroke is evident. Dementia usually presents later in the disease, with an average age of onset around 60 years, but a small percentage of these patients develop dementia in their thirties and forties (Chabriat & Bousser, 2007).

Magnetic resonance imaging (MRI) changes can be identified fairly early in the disease process and continue to progress as the disease progresses. Ischemic events develop several years after diagnosis, at age 40-50, although they can present earlier in many individuals with CADASIL. Ischemic events are present in up to 80% of individuals with CADASIL. This population is at a higher risk of seizure disorder, with up to 10% of people diagnosed with CADASIL having seizures. The majority of these individuals have seizures post-stroke.

Rarer symptoms of CADASIL include early onset of Parkinsonism (Van Gerpen, Ahlskog, & Petty, 2003), acute or sudden onset of deafness (Tournier-Lasserve, Iba-Zizen, Romero, & Bousser, 1991), and optic neuropathy (Rufa et al., 2004).

DIAGNOSIS
Genetic Testing
The most definitive test for diagnosis of CADASIL is genetic testing for the Notch 3 variant. Recent changes in genetic technologies have resulted in a decreased cost for genotyping. Many, but not all, insurance companies will cover the cost of genotyping. Genetic testing for the Notch 3 variant may be done using blood (white blood cells) or other tissues. Genetic testing, with or without positive results, can cause anxiety in patients and their family members. It is important that nurses caring for these patients are aware of the Genetic Information Non-discrimination Act (GINA) of 2008, which protects U.S. citizens from discrimination based on genetic information. In particular it provides protection against being denied insurance coverage, or discrimination in the workplace based on genetic information.

Skin Biopsy Testing
Skin biopsy with subsequent quantification of NOTCH3 protein product within the small vessels has also been utilized with adequate sensitivity and specificity. This test involves taking a small sample of skin and viewing the small blood vessels under electron microscopy. A positive test will show Granular Osmeophylic Material (GOM) and degeneration of the smooth muscle cell layer of vessels. The GOM creates lesions within the vessel that infiltrate the adventitial layer.

Radiographic Testing

Magnetic resonance imaging (MRI) will identify abnormal intensities associated with white matter lesions. T1 weighted images show hypointensities while T2 weighted images show hyperintensities in various white matter tracts. For the majority of CADASIL patients these findings occur together; however, in as many as 30%, only one of the two findings is present. T2 weighted hyperintensities are independently present, without T1 weighted hypointensities, in many early stage CADASIL patients, and they are common in asymptomatic children with the abnormal gene (Fattapposta et al., 2004). Abnormalities in the external capsule and anterior temporal lobe are fairly suggestive of CADASIL. MRI abnormalities may strongly suggest a diagnosis of CADASIL, but the patterns of abnormalities are also seen in other CNS disorders. Individuals with MRI abnormalities and symptoms suggesting CADASIL, particularly in the presence of family history of CADASIL or similar symptoms, should have follow-up genetic testing.

Genetic Counseling

CADASIL is a genetic disorder, and some form of counseling is generally appropriate. Genetic counseling may be necessary in select individuals. The majority of individuals with CADASIL have or had a parent with the disease. New mutations are rare, but counseling in combination with education on the disease may be helpful when they do occur. Individuals who had a parent die early in life, before symptoms of CADASIL would have appeared, may have inherited the gene without knowing they are at risk.

For parents, or individuals in their child-bearing years, counseling from a health care provider with specialized knowledge of genetic heritability of CADASIL is warranted. Genetic counselors and Genetic Nurse Counselors are health care professionals with training specific to the heritability patterns of genetic disorders/diseases and can assist these individuals in decision making. Generally, the risk of passing on the CADASIL variant gene is 50% for each pregnancy. Prenatal testing for the CADASIL variant is possible although rarely ordered for this adult-onset genetic disorder.

Psychological Counseling

While many of these health care professionals can also assist in the emotional challenges expressed with a diagnosis of CADASIL, psychiatric counseling may also be warranted.

PREVENTION OF ACUTE STROKE

While individuals with CADASIL are at high risk for stroke, they do not have many of the classic risk factors for stroke. It is difficult to promote lifestyle management in this population. Variation in the CADASIL gene, and specifically the abnormal version that leads to CADASIL pathology, is not correlated with symptom severity or development. Given that genetic variance is associated with development of CADASIL but not severity or speed of progression, it is likely that environmental factors significantly contribute to severity and progression of the disease. Specifically, smoking and elevated homocysteine levels contribute to severity and progression (Singhal, Bevan, Barrick, Rich, & Markus, 2004). Smoking cessation is strongly recommended to limit inflammatory response of the vessels and prevent further damage.

Individuals with CADASIL often have transient ischemic attacks (see Chapter 2) and multiple cerebral infarcts over the course of a lifetime. Treatment of patients with CADASIL is not curative and is focused primarily on limiting damage and maintaining optimal function. Antiplatelet agents (aspirin, clopidogrel, and aggrenox) have been used to decrease stroke frequency and thereby slow the progression of the disease. However, current research has not supported the efficacy of this practice (Hassan & Markus, 2000; Razvi, Davidson, Bone, & Muir, 2005). Angiography and anticoagulants are not recommended, as CADASIL is also associated with microvascular hemorrhage. Along these same lines, individuals with CADASIL presenting with acute stroke should not receive tPA due to the risk of hemorrhagic conversion.

MANAGING SYMPTOMS
Migraines

People with CADASIL are at increased risk for migraines, although the mechanism for this relationship is not clear. The frequency of migraine attacks is low in this population. There is minimal evidence suggesting superiority of any particular therapeutic.

Expert clinicians generally avoid ergot derivatives and trip-tans due to the strong vasoconstrictor effects and recommend non-steroidal anti-inflammatory drugs (Chabriat & Bousser, 2008; Chabriat, Joutel, Dichgans, Tournier-Lasserve, & Bousser, 2009) . Acetazolamide, a carbonic anhydrase inhibitor, is used to treat epilepsy and other neurologic disorders. Its efficacy in decreasing migraine burden in CADASIL has been reported in case studies only (Weller, Dichgans, & Klockgether, 1998; Forteza, Brozman, Rabinstein, Romano, & Bradley, 2001). Sodium valproate has been reported efficacious in some patients (Martikainen & Roine, 2012). Cessation of oral contraceptives may decrease frequency of migraines in women.

Cognitive decline
Donepezil is the only drug that has shown any efficacy in treating symptoms of CADASIL. In a randomized control trial of donepezil versus placebo in 161 patients, donepezil was shown to improve some measures of executive function but did not impact overall cognitive impairment (Dichgans et al., 2008).

REFERENCES
Buffon, F., Porcher, R., Hernandez, K., et al. (2006). Cognitive profile in CADASIL. *Journal of Neurology, Neurosurgery & Psychiatry*, *77*(2), 175–180.

Chabriat, H., & Bousser, M. G. (2007). Neuropsychiatric manifestations in CADASIL. *Dialogues in Clinical Neuroscience*, *9*(2), 199–208.

Chabriat, H., & Bousser, M. G. (2008). Cerebral autosomal dominant arteriopathy with subcortical infarcts and leukoencephalopathy. *Handbook of Clinical Neurology*, *89*, 671–686.

Chabriat, H., Joutel, A., Dichgans, M., Tournier-Lasserve, E., & Bousser, M. G. (2009). Cadasil. *Lancet Neurology*, *8*(7), 643–653.

Chabriat, H., Vahedi, K., Iba-Zizen, M. T., et al. (1995). Clinical spectrum of CADASIL: A study of 7 families. Cerebral autosomal dominant arteriopathy with subcortical infarcts and leukoencephalopathy. *Lancet*, *346*(8980), 934–939.

Desmond, D. W., Moroney, J. T., Lynch, T., Chan, S., Chin, S. S., & Mohr, J. P. (1999). The natural history of CADASIL: A pooled analysis of previously published cases. *Stroke*, *30*(6), 1230–1233.

Desmond, D. W., Tatemichi, T. K., Paik, M., & Stern, Y. (1993). Risk factors for cerebrovascular disease as correlates of cognitive function in a stroke-free cohort. *Archives of Neurology, 50*(2), 162–166.

Dichgans, M., Markus, H. S., Salloway, S., et al. (2008). Donepezil in patients with subcortical vascular cognitive impairment: a randomised double-blind trial in CADASIL. *Lancet Neurology, 7*(4), 310–318.

Dichgans, M., Mayer, M., Uttner, I., et al. (1998). The phenotypic spectrum of CADASIL: Clinical findings in 102 cases. *Annals of Neurology, 44*(5), 731–739.

Fattapposta, F., Restuccia, R., Pirro, C., et al. (2004). Early diagnosis in cerebral autosomal dominant arteriopathy with subcortical infarcts and leukoencephalopathy (CADASIL): The role of MRI. *Functional Neurology, 19*(4), 239–242.

Forteza, A. M., Brozman, B., Rabinstein, A. A., Romano, J. G., & Bradley, W. G. (2001). Acetazolamide for the treatment of migraine with aura in CADASIL. *Neurology, 57*(11), 2144–2145.

Hassan, A., & Markus, H. S. (2000). Genetics and ischaemic stroke. *Brain, 123*(9), 1784–1812.

Martikainen, M. H., & Roine, S. (2012). Rapid improvement of a complex migrainous episode with sodium valproate in a patient with CADASIL. *Journal of Headache & Pain, 13*(1), 95–97.

Razvi, S. S. M., Davidson, R., Bone, I., & Muir, K. W. (2005). Is inadequate family history a barrier to diagnosis in CADASIL? *Acta Neurologica Scandinavica, 112*(5), 323–326.

Rufa, A., De Stefano, N., Dotti, M. T., et al. (2004). Acute unilateral visual loss as the first symptom of cerebral autosomal dominant arteriopathy with subcortical infarcts and leukoencephalopathy. *Archives of Neurology, 61*(4), 577–580.

Singhal, S., Bevan, S., Barrick, T., Rich, P., & Markus, H. S. (2004). The influence of genetic and cardiovascular risk factors on the CADASIL phenotype. *Brain, 127*(9), 2031–2038.

Tournier-Lasserve, E., Iba-Zizen, M. T., Romero, N., & Bousser, M. G. (1991). Autosomal dominant syndrome with strokelike episodes and leukoencephalopathy. *Stroke, 22*(10), 1297–1302.

Vahedi, K., Chabriat, H., Levy, C., Joutel, A., Tournier-Lasserve, E., & Bousser M.-G. (2004). Migraine with aura and brain magnetic resonance imaging abnormalities in patients with CADASIL. *Archives of Neurology, 61*(8), 1237–1240.

Van Gerpen, J. A., Ahlskog, J. E., & Petty, G. W. (2003). Progressive supranuclear palsy phenotype secondary to CADASIL. *Parkinsonism & Related Disorders*, *9*(6), 367–369.

Verin, M., Rolland, Y., Landgraf, F., et al. (1995). New phenotype of the cerebral autosomal dominant arteriopathy mapped to chromosome 19: Migraine as the prominent clinical feature. *Journal of Neurology, Neurosurgery & Psychiatry*, *59*(6), 579–585.

Weller, M., Dichgans, J., & Klockgether, T. (1998). Acetazolamide-responsive migraine in CADASIL. *Neurology*, *50*(5), 1505.

Migraine Headache

9

Sheila A. Alexander

Evidence-Based Nursing Care for Stroke and Neurovascular Conditions,
First Edition. Edited by Sheila A. Alexander.
© 2013 John Wiley & Sons, Inc. Published 2013 by John Wiley & Sons, Inc.

Migraine headaches are recurring episodes of painful sensations that include throbbing and/or pulsing on one side of the head and are associated with nausea, vomiting, and sensitivity to light and/or sound. Migraines are often accompanied by an aura. Most auras associated with migraine headaches are visual in nature and include zig-zag lines, flashing lights, or a temporary loss of vision. Auras can also involve other sensory disturbances, speech disturbances, and motor function disturbances. Migraine headaches occur after exposure to a trigger in many individuals.

Migraines occur in about 12% of the Caucasian population and are three times more common in women as compared to men (Lipton et al., 2007). Migraine is ranked as the 19th leading cause of years living with disability in the general U.S. population and the 12th leading cause of years living with a disability in U.S. female population (Murthy et al., 2001). Migraines frequency is often progressive, with the most severe cases suffering migraines 15 or more days each month (Bigal & Lipton, 2006). Migraine clearly impairs functioning and quality of life during the actual headache attack, but sufferers of chronic migraines also report a decrease in quality of life outside these attacks. The significant impairment of function and quality of life during and in between migraine attacks warrants careful medical monitoring and acute and preventative treatment to minimize symptoms and improve quality of life. The overall goal of treatment of any patient with migraines should include prevention of attacks and acute relief of attacks through pharmacologic and/or nonpharmacologic means to restore maximum function and limit disability related to the disorder.

PATHOPHYSIOLOGY

Migraines often begin in childhood or early adulthood. In over 40% of migraine sufferers, migraines begin before the age of 18 (Bille, 1981). In industrialized countries, migraine is estimated to occur in up to 60% of children (Bille, 1981).

A single biological cause of migraine has not yet been identified and it is likely a multifactorial disorder, involving multiple genetic variants and multiple environmental exposures. It had been hypothesized that migraines were caused by dilation and constriction of cerebral blood vessels. Recent evidence suggests that migraines are more likely caused by abnormalities in neuronal cell function in distinct areas of the brain. Migraine with aura has been hypothesized to be caused by cortical spreading depression (CSD), a wave of neuronal activity followed by a period of neuronal inactivity that moves slowly across the cortex. The trigeminal nerve nuclei reside in the brainstem and innervate meningeal and superficial cortical blood vessels. Sensory stimulation of the trigeminal nerve nuclei are thought to also initiate brainstem activity sending pain signals up into the higher center of cortex. Recent animal studies have reported evidence that CSD activates the trigeminal nerve nuclei and initiate migraines.

Genetic studies have contributed significantly to advancement of the science in determining biological cause(s) of migraine with and without aura. Genes up-regulated or down-regulated before and during migraines or associated auras suggest possible biological pathways involved in their development and potential therapeutic targets. Additionally there is one form of migraine – familial hemiplegic migraine – that is inherited. Familial hemiplegic migraine is distinct from common migraine in that hemiplegia is common but other characteristics of migraine are also present. Given the heritable nature of this disorder, research has identified three associated genes – CACNA1A, ATP1A2, and SCN1A – that may also play a role in common migraine with or without aura. CACNA1A encodes an alpha-1 subunit of neuronal P/Q-type, voltage-gated calcium channels. ATP1A2 encodes the alpha-2 subunit of glial sodium-potassium pumps. SCN1A encodes the alpha-1 subunit of neuronal voltage-gated sodium channels. The association of these genetic variances with inherited migraine disorder suggests ion transportation alterations may be the cause of migraine symptoms.

The human methylenetretrahydrofolate reductase (MTHFR) gene on chromosome 1 produces a gene product that catalyses reactions [the nicotinamide adenine dinucleotide phosphate (NADPH) dependent conversion of 5, 10-methylenetetrahydrofolate (CH2-THF) to 5-methyltetrahydrofolate (CH3-THF), the circulatory form of folate and a cofactor for homocysteine methylation to methionone] for formation of circulatory folate and methionone (Goyette et al., 1994; Goyette et al., 1998). Circulatory homocysteine levels are upregulated in patients with migraine with aura, and it has been hypothesized that homocysteine acts as an excitatory amino acid, stimulating cerebral blood vessel vasodilation or temporary thrombosis of cerebral blood vessels, ultimately leading to a decrease in oxygen delivery to the brain and migraine (Kara, Sazci, Ergul, Kaya, & Kilic, 2003). Individuals with a specific genetic variant (C677T TT genotype) of the MTHFR gene have decreased MTHFR enzymatic activity and mild hyperhomocystinemia. Hyperhomocystinemia is pro-atherothrombotic and therefore can promote development of vascular disease, which may be involved in vascular-level changes that lead to mild hypoxia and migraine symptoms. Populations of individuals with migraine with aura more often have the MTHFR TT genotype (Kowa et al., 2000; Kara, Sazci, Ergul, Kaya, & Kilic, 2003; Lea et al., 2005; Scher et al., 2006). Specifically, the TT genotype has been associated with migraine with aura and unilateral head pain. The CT genotype has been associated with unilateral head pain, physical activity discomforts, and stress as a migraine trigger.

DIAGNOSIS
Diagnostic criteria
There is no biomarker or radiographic test available to diagnose migraines. As such, diagnosis is determined based on clinical presentation of symptoms. The International Headache Society has established criteria for diagnosing migraine headache disorders. There are two common forms of migraine: migraine with aura and migraine without aura. Migraine with aura is a debilitating, often bilateral headache lasting 4 to 72 hours. A prodromal or aura phase including transient focal symptoms, often of a visual nature, precedes the headache. Migraine without aura is a unilateral throbbing-type headache lasting up to 72 hours. Migraine without aura is aggravated by physical activity and accompanied by vomiting, nausea, photophobia and/or phonophobia, and signs of autonomic nervous system activation.

Assessment
There are many tools available to assess migraine frequency, intensity, and impact on quality of life.

The Migraine Prevention Questionnaire 5 (MPQ-5) is a tool used to evaluate severity and frequency of migraine while providing guidance in intervention (Lipton & Bigal, 2005, 2007). The patient provides the number of days in the past 1–3 months when they had a migraine, treated for migraine, and migraine affected activities. The summative score can be used to determine the efficacy of therapy or the need for preventive therapy.

The Headache Impact Test (HIT-6) is a six-question survey that evaluates impact of migraines on quality of life, by measuring time lost from daily activities due to migraine, pain severity, fatigue, and mood (Dowson, 2001).

The Migraine Disability Assessment (MIDAS) is a five-question self-administered survey that evaluates impact of migraine on quality of life, by assessing pain frequency, pain intensity, and reduced or missed activity in daily living situations (Stewart, Lipton, Kolodner, Liberman, & Sawyer, 1999).

There are other tools that measure the burden of migraine between attacks. These include the Migraine Interictal Burden Scale (MIBS), which measures the impact of migraine-related burden on work/school, family/social life, commitments/planning, and emotional/affective/cognitive distress. It is a four-item self-administered questionnaire designed for ease in clinical use, screening, and tracking changes over time.

Regardless of specific tools used to measure the impact of migraine on daily living, it is important to evaluate regularly and without judgment.

PREVENTING MIGRAINES
Identifying and avoiding triggers

Many sufferers of migraine headaches are aware of triggers or sensory exposures that initiate a migraine headache. For patients with known triggers, avoidance can prevent the onset of a migraine. Common triggers include exposure to bright light, flashing lights, sleep deprivation, and lack of food. Anxiety, stress, or relaxation can also serve as a trigger for a migraine headache. In women, migraines may be brought on by changes in hormone levels.

Tracking surroundings and a thorough history of the events for days before a migraine attack has been brought on can identify triggers. Patients should keep a diary of daily activities, hours of sleep, food and fluid intake, and emotions. Once a migraine has occurred, the time, date, intensity, and progression of symptoms should be recorded as well. A review of the diary considering potential trigger exposure for the minutes, hours, and then days before the migraine attack will highlight triggers. Triggers may then be avoided and migraines continuously monitored. Once a trigger, or perhaps a group of triggers, has been avoided, many patients will experience a significant decrease in frequency of migraines.

Exposure to bright lights or flashing lights is a relatively easy trigger to address. It is important to consider lighting when tracking migraine development. Hypoglycemia may be identified as a trigger that can be controlled with a regular healthy diet. Sleep deprivation is a trigger for some people. In this case, getting adequate sleep to prevent migraine for each individual is the goal. Stress and anxiety are potential triggers for migraine attacks that are difficult to control. Good stress management techniques may provide some relief.

Hormonal triggers are not avoidable, but knowledge of cyclical changes in hormones and how they initiate migraines may limit negative effects of migraines. For women who suffer migraines related to fluctuations in hormones at a given point in the menstrual cycle, it is possible to prophylactically treat potential migraines. Use of caffeine, ergot alkaloids, or other medications in development before symptoms begin may prevent the onset of migraine. Avoidance of other triggers during this high-risk periods may decrease frequency of migraines.

Antidepressants
Serotonin receptor antagonists
Serotonin receptors are found on cells in the CNS and peripheral nervous system (PNS). They bind with serotonin and facilitate neuronal transmission. When bound, serotonin receptors modify release of other neurotransmitters including gabba-amino-butyric acid (GABA), glutamate, dopamine, epinephrine, norepinephrine, and acetylcholine as well as hormone release. Drugs that modify serotonin receptor activity have been shown to decrease chronic pain of a variety of sorts, including migraine. Selective serotonin reuptake inhibitors (see Table 9.1 for the list) are typically used as antidepressants but also decrease frequency of migraine attacks for many sufferers. Selective serotonin reuptake inhibitors delay the uptake of serotonin by the pre-synaptic neuron from the synapse. Serotonin presence in the synapse enhances neuronal transmission, improving neuronal transmission and mediating symptoms.

Table 9.1 Serotonin receptor antagonists

Generic name	Common trade name(s)	Side effects
Citalopram	Celexa, Cipramil, Cipram, Dalsan, Recital, Emocal, Sepram, Seropram, Citox, Cital	Insomnia, drowsiness, apathy, emotional dampening, trembling, fatigue with excessive yawning, dry mouth, nausea, diarrhea, weight gain or loss, frequent urination, sweating, decreased libido, and anorgasmia.
		Less common but significant side effects include anxiety, dizziness, mood swings, headache, cardiac arrhythmia, blood pressure changes, vomiting, and bruxism. Rare but significant side effects include convulsions, hallucinations, and severe allergic reactions.
		*Contraindicated in patients taking monoamine oxidase inhibitors (MAOIs) or St. John's wort.
Escitalopram	Lexapro, Cipralex, Seroplex, Esertia	Insomnia, fatigue, somnolence, dizziness, akathisia, suicidality, dry mouth, diarrhea, constipation, sweating, indigestion, decreased libido, delayed ejaculation, and anorgasmia.
Fluoxetine	Prozac, Fontex, Seromex, Seronil, Sarafem, Ladose, Motivest	Insomnia, somnolence, nervousness, anxiety, dystonia, tardive dyskinesia, asthenia, tremor, mania, akathisia, vasculitis, lupus-like syndrome, rash, anorexia, nausea, anorgasmia, and decreased libido.
		*Contraindicated in patients taking monoamine oxidase inhibitors (MOAIs) or thioridazine.
Fluvoxamine	Luvox, Fevarin, Faverin, Dumyrox, Favoxil, Movox	Dizziness, nervousness, anxiety, paresthesias, headache, dry mouth, tachycardia, abdominal pain, nausea, vomiting, constipation, diarrhea, heartburn, loss of appetite, weight loss or gain, sweating, muscle weakness, drowsiness, difficulty sleeping, and unusual bruising.
Paroxetine	Paxil, Seroxat, Sereupin, Aropax, Deroxat, Divarius, Rexetin, Xetanor, Paroxat, Loxamine	Insomnia, agitation, mania, akathisia, somnolence, dizziness, tremor, paresthesias, memory problems, headache, dry mouth, nausea, weight gain, constipation, weakness, sweating, ejaculatory disturbance, male genital disorders.
Sertraline	Zoloft, Lustral, Serlain, Asentra	Insomnia, akathisia somnolence, dizziness, tremor, dry mouth, nausea, diarrhea, ejaculation failure, and decreased libido.
		*Contraindicated in patients taking monoamine oxidase inhibitors (MOAIs), pimozide, or disulfiram.
Ritanserin (serotonin antagonist)		

Tricyclic antidepressants

Research has shown that the use of certain tricyclic antidepressants may decrease frequency and severity of migraines. The use of these medications requires long-term commitment, as effects will not likely be seen until a therapeutic level has been reached, which can take one month or more. Consistent use over time leads to greater results. This class of drugs decreases the frequency but not the intensity of migraine attacks when compared to serotonin receptor antagonists. Side effects of Tricyclic antidepressants are also worth mentioning. Insomnia, sedation, dry mouth, and sexual dysfunction are common. See Table 9.2 for a list of tricyclic antidepressants and their efficacy and side effect profiles. Tricyclic antidepressants are used less often than serotonin receptor antagonists because fewer patients experience relief and side effects are more common and severe with use of a tricyclic antidepressant.

Anti-epileptics

Topiramate, valproic acid, and gabapentin are types of anti-epileptic medication used to treat migraine. These drugs can often decrease stress and anxiety, which in turn decreases trigger exposure, in addition to blocking the pathophysiologic pathway of migraine development. These drugs all target the serotonin system, and hence decrease migraine.

Behavioral therapies

Cognitive behavioral therapy is very effective in helping patients identify behaviors that trigger and/or lengthen the time of migraine headaches as well as non-therapeutic thoughts that decrease overall quality of life. This type of therapy can also be useful in treating depression, anxiety, panic disorder, and other co-morbidities common to patients with migraines. Cognitive behavioral therapy should only be administered by a trained and experienced professional.

Exercise can also help increase function in individuals affected with migraines. Exercise three times a week has been shown to decrease the frequency of migraines and intensity of symptoms, and to improve overall quality of life (Varkey, Cider, Carlsson, & Linde, 2009).

Table 9.2 Tricyclic antidepressants

Generic name	Common trade name	Side effects
Amitriptyline	Elavil, Tryptizol, Laroxyl, Sarotex, Lentizol	Nervousness, dizziness, insomnia, blurred vision, nausea, weight gain, appetite changes, nausea, constipation, dry mouth, urinary retention, and sexual dysfunction. Rare but significant side effects include confusion, seizures, mania, psychosis, depression, suicidal thoughts, extrapyramidal symptoms, feet or hand tingling/pain/numbness, sleep problems, hypnagogia, hypnopompia, tinnitus, cardiac arrhythmias, hypotension, heart block, painful/difficult urination, lip/oral ulcers, yellowing of the eyes and skin, breast tissue enlargement (males and females), abnormal breast milk production in females, and fever with sweating.
Maprotiline	Deprilept, Luidomil, Psymion	Dizziness, drowsiness, fatigue, agitation, confusion, mood swings, seizures, liver damage, leukopenia, agranulocytosis, dry mouth, increased appetite, weight gain, hypotension, tachycardia, cardiac arrhythmias, priapism, sexual dysfunction, photosensitivity of skin, and allergic skin reactions. Severe but rare side effects include polyneuritis, hepatitis, and erythema multiforme.

*Contraindicated in patients taking monoamine oxidase inhibitors (MAOIs). |
| Nortriptyline | Sensoval, Aventyl, Pamelor, Norpress, Allegron, Noritren and Nortrilen. | Sedation, dry mouth, rapid and irregular heart rate, increased appetite, constipation. Suicidal ideation in men more frequently than in women.

*Contraindicated in patients taking monoamine oxidase inhibitors (MAOIs). |
| Clomipramine | Anafranil | Fatigue, dizziness, lightheadedness, headaches, confusion, agitation, insomnia, nightmares, anxiety, seizures, hypotension, postural hypotension, arrhythmias, dry mouth, constipation, allergic skin reactions including photosensitivity, heartburn, weight gain, nausea, bruxism, sexual dysfunction in men.

Rare but significant side effects include hypomania, induction of schizophrenia, extrapyramidal side effects, ileus, liver damage, hepatitis, and leukopenia. |

(Continued)

Table 9.2 (Continued)

Generic name	Common trade name	Side effects
Mianserin	Bolvidon, Norval, Tolvon	Dizziness, seizures, sedation, drowsiness, somnolence, blurred vision, fainting, allergic reaction, agranulocytosis or white blood cell reduction, increased appetite, weight gain, dry mouth, and constipation.
Mirtazapine	Remeron, Avanza, Zispin	Dizziness, somnolence, sedation, malaise, vivid dreams/nightmares, blurry vision, dry mouth, increased appetite, weight gain, constipation, and enhanced libido.
		Less common but significant side effects include agitation/restlessness, irritability, aggression, apathy, calmness, anhedonia, difficulty swallowing, shallow breathing, low body temperature, loss of balance, restless legs syndrome, nocturnal emissions, spontaneous orgasm, and, in some patients, mild hallucinogenic effects.
		Very rare but significant side effects include allergic reaction, edema, fainting, seizures, bone marrow suppression, myelodysplasia, and agranulocytosis.
Doxepin – also has anxiolytic properties	Aponal, Adapine, Deptran, Sinquan, Sinequan, Silenor	Fatigue, dizziness, drowsiness, lightheadedness, confusion, nightmares, agitation, anxiety, insomnia, delirium, tinnitus, dry mouth, obstipation, difficulty urinating, sweating, precipitation of glaucoma, hypotension, postural hypotension, arrhythmias, skin rash, skin photosensitivity, increased appetite, weight gain, and impaired sexual function in men.
		Less common but significant side effects include seizures, hypomania, schizophrenia, extrapyramidal symptoms, nausea, ileus, leukopenia, thrombopenia, agranulocytosis, hypoplastic anemia, liver damage, hepatitis, hypertension, polyeuropathy, and breast enlargement and galactorrhea in both males and females.
Desipramine	Norpramin, Pertofane	Dysrhythmias, sudden cardiac death.

Relaxation therapy can aid many patients in decreasing the physiologic response to stress, which may decrease the frequency of migraines. Typical methods include diaphragmatic breathing, visual imagery, prayer, meditation, self-hypnosis, guided relaxation CDs/tapes, or yoga. Relaxation requires a commitment, because all of these methods require regular practice for maximal efficacy. While relaxation therapy is often initially administered by a trained health care professional, patients are able to practice independently and can train themselves through the use of commercially available training manuals, audio recordings, or visual relaxation aids.

Biofeedback is a method for patients to become aware of involuntary physiologic functions and bring them under voluntary control to decrease symptoms. Using this method, patients learn to identify and control some symptoms, particularly those related to sympathetic stimulation, including improved circulation and decreased muscle tension, which may decrease the frequency and/or intensity of migraine attacks. Biofeedback should only be administered by a trained and experienced professional.

TREATING MIGRAINES
Environmental
Much like when avoiding triggers, modifying the environment can serve to decrease the intensity of a migraine and make the sufferer less uncomfortable. A quiet, dark room with minimal or no light may alleviate some symptoms of migraine.

Medications
Simple analgesics
Simple analgesics can often provide relief from symptoms and, if effective, should be used as first-line therapy. Aspirin, acetaminophen, and non-steroidal anti-inflammatory drugs (NSAIDS) can be purchased without prescription and are easily available to most patients. Many patients with migraines will have already tried one or more of these agents, and failed therapies should be considered during treatment planning. During intial treatment planning, a thorough assessment of remedies attempted and their success should be completed. If an individual has obtained relief with one agent, such as aspirin, that therapy should be continued if not contraindicated by co-morbidities. If one agent has been used without

---

success, a repeat trial is not likely to yield success, but a different agent might, in particular one with a different mechanism of action.

After cell damage, phospholipids in the cell membrane release arachadonic acid, intiating a cascade of events resulting in prostaglandin and thromboxane production. Prostaglandins regulate smooth muscle contraction and relaxation, modify platelet aggregation, decrease gastric acid secretion, increase gastric mucus secretion, stimulate the thermoregulatory center of the hypothalmus to produce fever, and sensitize spinal neurons to pain. Thromboxane facilitates platelet aggregation and causes vasoconstriction. Aspirin inactivates cyclooxygenase, the enzyme that converts arachadonic acid to prostaglandins and thromboxanes, thereby decreasing pain.

Acetaminophen is an analgesic without a clear mechanism of action. Acetaminophen likely inhibits cyclooxygenase activity but is somewhat specific to the cyclooxygenase 2 subtype and has CNS effects not present in aspirin or NSAIDS. The selective inhibition of cyclooxygenase-2 results in prostaglandin, but not thromboxane, inhibition. Current research suggests that acetaminophen also decreases pain by modulating the endogenous cannabinoid system in the CNS (Hogestatt et al., 2005).

NSAIDS are a class of drugs with anti-inflammatory, and therefore analgesic and antipyretic, actions. Most NSAIDS are general cyclooxygenase inhibitors, acting on both cyclooxygenase 1 and cyclooxygenase 2.

Many patients have experience with these medications for migraines and other types of pain. It is important to consider the patients previous experience and successes with each medication. If use of one of these analgesics does not provide adequate relief, addition of an anti-emetic or other combination of medications may lead to success.

Anti-emetic agents
Anti-emetics provide relief when given in combination with analgesics.

Caffeine
Caffeine is an adenosine receptor antagonist. Upon caffeine binding to the adenosine receptor, the receptor is occupied but not activated.

Caffeine has vasoconstrictor effects that are thought to be the mechanism of action in treating migraines. Caffeine is most effective in combination with other medications such as aspirin, NSAIDs, or ergot alkaloids.

Ergot alkaloids

Ergot alkaloids naturally occur in fungi and select plants. They induce vasoconstriction within the human body and in this way decrease symptoms of migraine. The structure of ergot alkaloids is similar to many neurotransmitters including serotonin, dopamine, and epinephrine, and as such can bind to many receptors within the CNS.

Ergotamine specifically binds with the 5HT1B serotonin receptor, causing vasoconstriction, and with the 5HT10 serotonin receptor, inhibiting trigeminal nerve activity. Significant side effects are common with ergotamine use, which limits their use for treatment of migraine. Ergotamine also binds with D2 dopamine receptors and 5HT1A receptors, leading to significant side effects. Common side effects include gastrointestinal irritability, peripheral tingling, angina, drowsiness, dizziness, and rebound headaches. The superior efficacy of triptans in combination with these significant side effects has led to decreased use of ergotamine.

Dihydroergotamine binds with dopamine and adrenergic receptors in addition to 5HT2B and 5HT2C receptors. It has significantly fewer side effects so it is a more appealing treatment option than ergotamine. Due to poor oral bioavailability, and a lack of general availability of the oral form, this drug is not given orally in the United States. It is available in intranasal, subcutaneous, intramuscular, and/or intravenous injection forms. The intranasal form has 32A% bioavailability compared to the other forms. Intravenous injection is extremely effective but often produces nausea. Nausea can by controlled with prophylactic anti-emetics. It is important to note that Dihydroergotamine should not be administered within 24 hours of triptans due to the strong vasoconstrictor effects.

Triptans bind with 5HT1B and 5HT10 receptors and thus have similar actions to ergotamine. The higher efficacy of triptans in relieving acute migraine headache is likely due to broader binding activity. Triptans act on nerve endings, blocking release of pain-modifying peptides, as well as on blood vessels and therefore have a dual mechanism for blocking pain impulses. It is important to note that triptans have strong vasoconstrictive activity and should not be given with other drugs inducing strong vasoconstriction due to the risk of coronary artery vasopasm.

Steroids

A single dose of dexamethasone in combination with standard treatment has been associated with a decrease in headache frequency (Coleman et al., 2008).

Medications in development

Ginkgolide B is an herbal treatment used with some success in treating migraines. It is a known anti-platelet-activating factor that promotes inflammation and stimulates nociceptive agent. Ginkgolide B has been shown to decrease frequency of headaches in children and young adults (Usai, Grazzi, Andrasik, & Bussone, 2010). Ginkgolide B modulates glutamate activity in such a manner that decreases glutamate and aura. Abnormal glutamate levels have been associated with migraine aura. Platelet-activating factor is also released during the aura phase of migraine, leading to trigeminal nerve sensitization and pain.

Metoprolol (Lopressor and Toprol-XL) is a selective beta 1 receptor blocker that has been used in the treatment of migraine. It is associated with the following side effects: bradycardia, fainting, dizziness, lightheadedness, drowsiness, tiredness, mood changes, depression, unusual dreams, ataxia, difficulty sleeping, vision problems, increased thirst, shortness of breath, coughing, dyslipidemia, cold or numb hands and feet, blue fingers and toes, numbness/tingling of the hands or feet, diarrhea, erectile dysfunction, sexual dysfunction, and hair loss. Less common but significant side effects include easy bruising/bleeding, persistent sore throat, persistent fever, yellowing of skin or eyes, stomach pain, dark urine, and persistent nausea.

Propranolol is a nonselective beta blocker that relieves symptoms in some migraine sufferers. Trade names include Inderal, Inderal LA, Avlocardyl, Deralin, Dociton, Inderalici, InnoPran XI, Sumial, Anaprilinum, and Bedranol SR.

Buspirone is a piperazine and azapirone class drug used primarily as an anxiolytic that has been used in combination with tricyclic antidepressants to treat migraine. It is a 5HT1A receptor partial agonist, D2 dopamine receptor antagonist, and alpha1 and alpha2 adrenergic receptor antagonist.

Diazepam is a benzodiazepine derivative used to treat many disorders, as well as during medical procedures. It has anxiolytic, anticonvulsant, hypnotic sedative, skeletal muscle relaxant, and amnestic properties. It binds to a specific site on gamma-amino-butyric acid receptors and leads to general CNS depression. Adverse effects include anterograde amnesia, sedation, paradoxical effects (excitement, rage, seizures in some epileptics), and depression. It is rarely used to treat migraines due to addictive qualities of this drug.

Appropriate use of medications to treat migraines is important to avoid side effects and, in certain situations, addiction. Proper use of acute medications, in combination with preventative strategies, will provide a consistent decrease in frequency and severity of headaches. Overuse of acute medications can lead to tolerance and decrease in efficacy. Assessment of patients using acute medications should be done at each office visit to determine effectiveness of pain control and evaluation overuse. Buse, Rupnow, and Lipton (2009, p. 429) provide an excellent series of questions to routinely evaluate medication overuse:

1. Do you ever take a pill before social events or work meetings or because you are anxious before migraine symptoms start?
2. Do you ever take a pill just in case?
3. Do you use acute treatment three or more days a week?
4. In addition to your prescription medications, about how often do you take over-the-counter pain medications?

ADDITIONAL RESOURCES

Headache Impact Test-6 Web site. http://www.headachetest.com/HIT6/PDFS/English.pdf. Accessed January 13, 2009.

Ramadan, N. M., Silberstein, S. D., Freitag, F. G., Gilbert, T. T., & Frishberg, B. M. (2009). U.S. Headache Consortium. Evidence-based guidelines for migraine headache in the primary care setting: pharmacological management for prevention of migraine. http://www.aan.com/professionals/practice/pdfs/gl0090.pdf. Accessed January 13, 2009.

Schurks, M. et al. (2008). Interrelationships among the MTHFR 677C>T polymorphism, migraine, and cardiovascular disease. *Neurology*, *71*(7), 505–513.

Ware Jr., J. E., Bjorner, J. B., & Kosinski, M. (2000). Practical implications of item response theory and computerized adaptive testing: A brief summary of ongoing studies of widely used headache impact scales. *Medical Care*, *38*(9)(Suppl), II73–II82.

World Health Organization. (2001). *The World Health Report 2001: Mental Health: New Understanding, New Hope*. [2]l. Accessed January 12, 2009.

REFERENCES

Bigal, M. E., & Lipton, R. B. (2006). When migraine progresses: transformed or chronic migraine. *Expert Review of Neurotherapeutics*, *6*(3), 297–306.

Bille, B. (1981). Migraine in childhood and its prognosis. *Cephalalgia*, *1*(2), 71–75.

Buse, D. C., Rupnow, M. F. T., & Lipton, R. B. (2009). Assessing and managing all aspects of migraine: Migraine attacks, migraine-related functional impairment, common comorbidities, and quality of life. *Mayo Clinic Proceedings*, *85*(5), 422–435.

Colman, I., Friedman, B. W., Brown, M. D., et al. (2008). Parenteral dexamethasone for acute severe migraine headache: Meta-analysis of randomised controlled trials for preventing recurrence. *British Medical Journal*, *336*(7657), 1359–1361.

Dowson, A. J. (2001). Assessing the impact of migraine. *Current Medical Research & Opinion*, *17*(4), 298–309.

Goyette, P., Pai, A., Milos, R., et al. (1998). Gene structure of human and mouse methylenetetrahydrofolate reductase (MTHFR). [Erratum appears in *Mammalian Genome* (1999), *10*(2), 204]. *Mammalian Genome*, *9*(8), 652–656.

Goyette, P., Sumner, J. S., Milos, R., et al. (1994). Human methylenetetrahydrofolate reductase: isolation of cDNA, mapping and mutation identification.[Erratum appears in *Nature Genetics* (1994), *7*(4), 551]. *Nature Genetics*, *7*(2), 195–200.

Hogestatt, E. D., Jonsson, B. A. G., Ermund, A., et al. (2005). Conversion of acetaminophen to the bioactive N-acylphenolamine AM404 via fatty acid amide hydrolase-dependent arachidonic acid conjugation in the nervous system. *Journal of Biological Chemistry*, *280*(36), 31405–31412.

Kara, I., Sazci, A., Ergul, E., Kaya, G., & Kilic, G. (2003). Association of the C677T and A1298C polymorphisms in the 5,10 methylenetetrahydrofolate reductase gene in patients with migraine risk. *Brain Research*, *111*(1–2), 84–90.

Kowa, H., Yasui, K., Takeshima, T., Urakami, K., Sakai, F., & Nakashima, K. (2000). The homozygous C677T mutation in the methylenetetrahydrofolate reductase gene is a genetic risk factor for migraine. *American Journal of Medical Genetics*, *96*(6), 762–764.

Lea, R. A., Ovcaric, M., Sundholm, J., Solyom, L., Macmillan, J., & Griffiths, L. R. (2005). Genetic variants of angiotensin converting enzyme and methylenetetrahydrofolate reductase may act in combination to increase migraine susceptibility. *Brain Research*, *136*(1–2), 112–117.

Lipton, R. B., & Bigal, M. E. (2005). Migraine: Epidemiology, impact, and risk factors for progression. *Headache*, *45*(Suppl 1), S3–S13.

Lipton, R. B., & Bigal, M. E. (2007). Ten lessons on the epidemiology of migraine. *Headache*, *47*(Suppl 1), S2–S9.

Lipton, R. B., Bigal, M. E., Diamond, M., et al. (2007). Migraine prevalence, disease burden, and the need for preventive therapy. *Neurology*, *68*(5), 343–349.

Murthy, R. S., Bertolote, J. M., Epping-Jordan, J., et al. (2001). *The World health report: 2001: Mental health: New understanding, new hope*. Geneva: World Health Organization.

Scher, A. I., Terwindt, G. M., Verschuren, W. M. M., et al. (2006). Migraine and MTHFR C677T genotype in a population-based sample. *Annals of Neurology*, *59*(2), 372–375.

Stewart, W. F., Lipton, R. B., Kolodner, K., Liberman, J., & Sawyer, J. (1999). Reliability of the migraine disability assessment score in a population-based sample of headache sufferers. *Cephalalgia*, *19*(2), 107–114; discussion on p. 114.

Usai, S., Grazzi, L., Andrasik, F., & Bussone, G. (2010). An innovative approach for migraine prevention in young age: A preliminary study. *Neurological Sciences*, *31*(Suppl 1), S181–S183.

Varkey, E., Cider, A., Carlsson, J., & Linde, M. (2009). A study to evaluate the feasibility of an aerobic exercise program in patients with migraine. *Headache*, *49*(4), 563–570.

Moyamoya Disease

10

Sheila A. Alexander

Evidence-Based Nursing Care for Stroke and Neurovascular Conditions,
First Edition. Edited by Sheila A. Alexander.
© 2013 John Wiley & Sons, Inc. Published 2013 by John Wiley & Sons, Inc.

Moyamoya disease is a condition of bilateral intracerebral internal carotid artery stenosis that increases risk of hypoxia and ischemic stroke. Moyamoya syndrome refers to the presence of unilateral Moyamoya vascular malformation or unilateral or bilateral Moyamoya vascular malformation in combination with head/neck radiotherapy, Down syndrome, neurofibromatosis, and sickle cell disease. Less frequently, Moyamoya vascular anomalies have been associated with congenital cardiac anomalies, renal artery stenosis, hyperthyroidism, and giant cervicofacial hemangiomas. The hallmarks of Moyamoya disease are cerebral vessel constriction leading to obstruction and subsequent development of collateral flow through small, weak vessels that are prone to leakage. The internal carotid arteries are most commonly involved. The internal lumen of the affected arteries is decreased, causing a decrease in blood flow to brain tissue. Collateral blood vessels form to compensate for the decreased blood flow, but the newly formed vessels are dilated, smaller, and weaker than the original arteries.

Moyamoya is a Japanese word that loosely translates as "puff of smoke." The name describes the appearance of the dilated collateral blood vessels that develop when the internal carotid artery and sometimes the middle cerebral artery and anterior cerebral arteries are blocked.

Moyamoya disease affects children and adults, although there are typically different presentations for children compared to adults. Children with Moyamoya typically present around 5 years of age with strokes, with ischemic stroke being more common, or transient ischemic attacks. Headaches are common, often associated with crying, coughing, straining, or exercise. Progressive cognitive decline, seizures, dizziness, vision problems, sensory impairment, hemiparesis, monoparesis, and involuntary arm or leg movement are common symptoms.

Adults typically present with Moyamoya in their mid-thirties to mid-forties with acute hemorrhagic or ischemic stroke (Soriano, Sethna, & Scott, 1993; Guzman et al., 2009). While ischemic stroke is more common, hemorrhagic stroke can also occur in people with Moyamoya. The collateral vessels that form in response to the decreased cerebral blood flow are weak and prone to hemorrhage (Han, Nam, & Oh, 1997; Wakai et al., 1997; Han et al., 2000; Baba, Houkin, & Kuroda, 2008). Hemorrhagic stroke typically occurs in the deep diencephalon regions of the brain, including the basal ganglia, thalamus, and ventricular wall. Non-traumatic acute subdural hematoma may also occur due to rupture of fragile collateral vessels in that area. Transient ischemic attack, seizures, convulsions, and migraine-like attacks are common.

Moyamoya is more common in people of Asian descent, and most common in the Japanese, with an overall incidence of 0.54/100,000 in that country (Kuriyama et al., 2008). In the North American population, the incidence is .086/100,000 (Uchino, Johnston, Becker, & Tirschwell, 2005). Moyamoya is more common in women than men (1.8:1) (Kuriyama et al., 2008).

Prognosis of untreated Moyamoya is very poor, with major deficit or mortality occurring in about 75% of patients within 2 years of diagnosis. With proper treatment to prevent brain tissue ischemia and damage, the morbidity and mortality rates approach normal for the age group of the patient.

PATHOPHYSIOLOGY

Moyamoya is caused by progressive intima medial thickening of the artery, hyperplasia of smooth muscle cells decreasing the internal lumen of the artery and promoting clot formation. The intracranial portion of the internal carotid artery is a common site of blockage, but the anomaly often extends into the middle cerebral arteries and anterior cerebral arteries.

Prolonged inflammation also has been implicated as a mediating factor of Moyamoya disease development, primarily due to one large study showing over 60% of people with Moyamoya disease had pre-existing inflammatory disease. While a causative role has not been identified, fibroblast growth factor (Houkin, Ishikawa, Kuroda, & Abe, 1998), soluble vascular-cell adhesion molecule type 1, intercellular adhesion molecule type 1, and E-selectin are all elevated in the cerebrospinal fluid of people with Moyamoya disease (Soriano, Cowan, Proctor, & Scott, 2002). These findings suggest central nervous system inflammation and blood brain barrier dysfunction. Increased endothelial progenitor cells are also present, suggesting angiogenesis and arteriogenesis (Mineharu et al., 2008). Additional mechanisms implicated in Moyamoya disease include caspase-dependent apoptosis, direct vessel injury, immunologic targeting of vascular tissue, select infectious processes, and radiation (Inoue, Ikezaki, Sasazuki, Matsushima, & Fukui, 2000; Takagi, Kikuta, Sadamasa, Nozaki, & Hashimoto, 2006a, 2006b; Longo et al., 2008).

There is evidence that Moyamoya is caused by a genetic mutation. A section on the long arm of chromosome 17 (Mineharu et al., 2008) and on chromosome 6 (Inoue et al., 2000) have been implicated. The incidence of Moyamoya in select Japanese families is as high as 7%, suggesting that genetic variation may be driving the abnormal vessel development. Additionally, patients with select genetic diseases, including neurofibromatosis, Down syndrome, and sickle cell disease, have a higher rate of Moyamoya.

Cerebral aneurysms are common in patients with Moyamoya disease. The exact mechanism driving this relationship is not clear. Two potential hypotheses suggest that aneurysms form due to the increased stress in the abnormally dilated vessels or that genetic/congenital defect in artery formation promotes both Moyamoya and aneurysm formation.

Autopsy reports have informed knowledge of the altered physiology of Moyamoya. Increased intima media thickening with and without lipid deposition and edema, thinning or duplication of the intima media layer, media and adventitia thinning, and fibrin deposition within the wall have all been found on autopsy of patients with Moyamoya.

DIAGNOSIS

A number of radiographic tests can identify Moyamoya. The distinct vascular features are seen on CT scan, MRI, and angiogram.

Conventional angiography is the gold standard for diagnosis of Moyamoya. This technique provides optimal visualization of the actual vessels involved and newly developed collateral flow. It should be performed in the operative planning phase as it generates data that can be used to determine approach and surgical procedure. Moyamoya disease is categorized based on angiographic findings. Presence of collateral vessels and increased vessel occlusion indicate increased disease burden and progression (see Tables 10.1 and 10.2).

T1 weighted images show the vascular anomalies more clearly than FLAIR images.

Table 10.1 Moyamoya classification based on angiography

	Angiographic findings
Grade I	Carotid stenosis, no collateral vessels
Grade II	Basal collateral vessels
Grade III	Prominent collateral vessels
Grade IV	Stenotic or occluded vessel(s) of the Circle of Willis and posterior cerebral arteries
Grade V	Extracranial collateral network
Grade VI	Total carotid occlusion

Created from information in Suzuki, J., & Takaka, A. (1969). Cerebrovascular "moyamoya" disease: Disease showing abnormal net-like vessels in base of brain. *Archives of Neurology, 20,* 288–299.

MRI and MRA are most commonly used for the diagnosis and monitoring of Moyamoya. Diffusion-weighted imaging is commonly used in children.

Xenon-enhanced computed tomography (XeCT), transcranial doppler ultrasonography, positive emission tomography (PET), and single-photon emission computed tomography (SPECT) imaging are less frequently used to diagnose Moyamoya disease and are used to monitor cerebral blood flow and oxygen supply to brain tissue.

Table 10.2 Suzuki grading system

Grading	Definition
Grade I	Narrowing of ICA apex
Grade II	Initiation of moyamoya collaterals
Grade III	Progressive ICA stenosis with intensification of moyamoya-associated collaterals.
Grade IV	Development of ECA collaterals
Grade V	Intensification of ECA collaterals and reduction of moyamoya-associated collaterals.
Grade VI	Total occlusion of ICA and disappearance of moyamoya-associated collaterals.

MEDICAL TREATMENT

Medical management of Moyamoya disease can be used to alleviate symptoms but does not alter disease progression. The stroke risk associated with medical management of symptoms of Moyamoya disease without surgical intervention is high, ranging from 65% to 85% depending on the number of vessels involved (Baaj et al., 2009).

Aspirin or ticlopidine may be used to decrease coagulation, promoting improved blood flow to the brain. Calcium channel blockers or pentoxifylline may be used to induce vasodilation. Anticonvulsants should be used for seizure control as needed.

A thorough assessment of symptoms and symptom history should occur. Events that precipitate symptoms, particularly symptoms of transient ischemic attacks, may be identified and avoidance techniques may be developed. People with Moyamoya disease should not participate in activities with a high risk of traumatic brain injury to avoid potentially complicating events. This can be particularly concerning for children and adolescents. Parents of children newly diagnosed with Moyamoya disease have increased anxiety and concerns regarding the progressive nature of the disease, the inheritability of the disease, symptoms, developmental delays, and surgical management procedures. Fear of seizures and social isolation has also been reported. Support and sometimes psychological counseling should be provided to both the patient and the family. Genetic counseling should be provided to patients and their families. Genetic counseling can aid in decision making regarding risk of passing on a genetic disorder and family planning.

SURGICAL TREATMENTS

Surgical treatments are available for treatment of Moyamoya disease. Revascularization surgery is a common treatment for Moyamoya disease. Blood vessels are either moved to provide blood flow to at-risk brain tissue or placed against the brain tissue to promote angiogenesis – the formation of new blood vessels. The decision to perform surgery must consider the overall health of the patient, the symptom history, and radiography findings.

Patients with a history of ischemic symptoms or hemorrhagic stroke are good surgical candidates. Progressive cognitive decline or frequent/progressive seizures warrants consideration of surgical procedures.

Preoperative care

Preoperative assessment is similar to other cerebral neurosurgeries. Medical history, laboratory values, co-morbidities, and previous cerebrovascular events should be considered.

Cerebral angiography must be performed to determine the approach and extent of the surgical procedure. Angiograms should visualize the internal carotid arteries, external carotid arteries, vertebral arteries, and middle cerebral and anterior cerebral arteries if involved. Angiographic results show the size of the malformation, location of the malformation, as well as the size and location of vessels to be used for revascularization.

Cerebral blood flow studies are routinely performed preoperatively. XeCT is a common method.

Severe anemia should be reversed before surgery to optimize oxygen-carrying capacity.

For patients taking anticonvulsants and/or calcium channel blockers preoperatively, these should be continued until the day of surgery. Aspirin therapy should be discontinued 7–10 days before surgery and is often safely replaced with low-molecular-weight heparin.

NPO status should be maintained after midnight before surgery. Many facilities admit patients with Moyamoya disease the evening before surgery (Smith & Scott, 2005). This permits intravenous hydration, decreasing dehydration that contributes to decreased cerebral blood flow.

Anxiolytics are commonly administered preoperatively. This is particularly useful in children as crying causes hyperventilation, which can result in hypocapnia and cerebral blood flow alterations. No specific anxiolytics have been studied to determine efficacy.

Operative procedures

Direct revascularization surgery connects an external scalp artery to the internal artery that is problematic (the internal carotid and/or middle cerebral artery). Superficial temporal artery–middle cerebral artery or external carotid artery–middle cerebral artery bypass are the most common direct revascularization surgeries to treat Moyamoya. The small size of the vessels in children makes this a difficult procedure. Complications of direct revascularization surgery include arterial occlusion, blood pressure fluctuation, hyperemia, and seizures (Miyamoto, Akiyama, & Nagata, 1998; Fujimara, Mugikura, & Kaneta, 2008). There is a 4% risk of stroke after surgery (Scott & Smith, 2009).

Indirect revascularization surgery modifies blood vessels so that they lie against the brain tissue at risk, promoting new vessel formation.

Encephaloduroarteriosynangiosis (EDAS) is a procedure commonly used to treat Moyamoya disease. This procedure requires surgical displacement of the skin over the scalp, dissection of a large section of a superficial temporal artery, removal of a small portion of the bone and dura, and attachment of the superficial temporal artery to dural opening before the bone is replaced. The superficial temporal artery will spawn new blood vessels to adequately perfuse the brain at risk over the months following this procedure. Because the scalp artery is modified and attached to the dural opening, once this procedure has been completed, it is not possible to perform the superficial temporal artery–middle cerebral artery bypass surgery. Pial synangiosis is a similar procedure. The skin and skull over the surgical area are displaced, the arachnoid tissue is removed, and the posterior branch of the superficial temporal artery is attached to the pial surface, promoting new collateral blood vessel formation.

Encephalomyosynangiosis (EMS) is a procedure where the skin over the temporalis muscle is displaced, the temporalis muscle is dissected, bone is removed, and a portion of the muscle is attached to the brain tissue before replacing the bone. The muscle tissue will spawn angiogenesis.

Encephalomyoarteriosynangiosis (EMAS) is a procedure combining EDAS and EMS.

Encephaloduroarteriosynangiosis (EDAMS) is a similar procedure combining aspects of other indirect revascularization procedures. EDAMS involves placement of a portion of the temporalis muscle, a segment of the superficial temporal artery, and a section of the galeal flap, which are secured together and attached to the dura against the ischemic brain tissue in an effort to stimulate revascularization.

Multiple burrholes may be created as a single procedure or in combination with one of the above procedures to stimulate new blood vessel growth from the scalp into the brain tissue.

In general, direct revascularization procedures are difficult to perform in children due to the small size of the involved vessels. Children have a higher rate of neoangiogenesis after indirect revascularization procedures, making these a more attractive treatment.

Overall, the success rate for symptom relief after direct and indirect revascularization is 87% (Fung, Thompson, & Ganesan 2005). The 5 year stroke risk after revascularization is 5.6%, compared to 65.7% in Moyamoya disease patients not treated with revascularization (Guzman et al., 2009).

Intra-operative care

The anesthesia needs are different for patients, and children in particular, with Moyamoya disease requiring surgery. The overall goal is to maintain the balance between oxygen supply and demand during the procedure. Hypotension and increased cerebral oxygen metabolism should be avoided and normocarbia should be maintained. Blood pressure should be maintained at or above preoperative levels to promote adequate cerebral perfusion. Fluid loss should be carefully monitored and replaced during surgery to prevent hypotension and inadequate cerebral perfusion. Evidence suggests Moyamoya disease patients should be maintained in a hypervolemic state during revascularization procedures. Hypercapnia should be avoided to prevent ischemia and infarction.

It is important to monitor neurologic status throughout the procedure. Different facilities use different methods, but electroencephalography, somatosensory evoked potentials, transcranial doppler ultrasonography, and near-infrared spectroscopy have been reported useful (Baykan, Ozgen, Ustalar, Dagcinar, & Ozek, 2005; Smith & Scott, 2005). There is no evidence supporting the use of transcranial doppler ultrasonography or near-infrared spectroscopy for early detection of infarction or improved outcomes after revascularization surgery.

Temperature control should be actively supported during the operative phase. Hypothermia should be considered, although

there is minimal empirical evidence suggesting its efficacy compared to normothermia. Hyperthermia should be avoided due to the resultant increase in cerebral metabolic rate.

Post-operative care

In the early post-operative phase, imaging should be ordered to determine bypass patency, revascularization extent, and affected vessel regression. Cerebral angiography is most commonly used, but magnetic resonance angiography is being used with increased frequency. Cerebral blood flow studies are used to assess improvement in perfusion.

Blood pressure should be maintained at or above preoperative levels to prevent ischemia or infarct. Fluid status should be closely monitored and fluid replacement should be administered to maintain a euvolemic or slight hypervolemic state to prevent hypovolemia and resultant decreases in cerebral perfusion for 48–72 hours.

Pain should be controlled tightly in the post-operative phase to decrease crying, neuroendocrine response, and the increase in cerebral metabolism that promotes infarction.

Aspirin may be restarted 24 hours post-operatively. Anticonvulsants should be continued.

Occupational therapy, physical therapy, and speech therapy should be employed as needed to maximize functional recovery, particularly in patients with deficits from stroke.

REFERENCES

Baaj, A. A., Agazzi, S., Sayed, Z. A., Toledo, M., Spetzler, R. F., & van Loveren, H. (2009). Surgical management of moyamoya disease: A review. *Neurosurgical Focus*, *26*(4), E7.

Baba, T., Houkin, K., & Kuroda, S. (2008). Novel epidemiological features of moyamoya disease. *Journal of Neurology, Neurosurgery & Psychiatry*, *79*(8), 900–904.

Baykan, N., Özgen, S., Ustalar, Z. S., Dagcinar, A., & Ozek, M. M. (2005). Moyamoya disease and anesthesia. *Paediatric Anaesthesia*, *15*(12), 1111–1115.

Fujimara, M., Mugikura, S., & Kaneta, T. (2008). Incidence and risk factors for symptomatic cerebral hyperperfusion after superficial

termporal artery-middle cerebral artery anastomosis in patients with moyamoya disease. *Surgical Neurology*, *71*, 223–227.

Fung, L., Thompson, D., & Ganesan, V. (2005). Revascularisation surgery for pediatric moyamoya: A review of literature. *Children's Nervous Systems*, *21*, 358–364.

Guzman, R., Lee, M., Achrol, A., et al. (2009). Clinical outcome after 450 revascularization procedures for moyamoya disease. Clinical article. *Journal of Neurosurgery*, *111*(5), 927–935.

Han, D. H., Kwon, O. K., Byun, B. J., et al. (2000). A co-operative study: clinical characteristics of 334 Korean patients with moyamoya disease treated at neurosurgical institutes (1976–1994). The Korean Society for Cerebrovascular Disease. *Acta Neurochirurgica*, *142*(11), 1263–1273; discussion on pp. 1263–1264.

Han, D. H., Nam, D. H., & Oh, C. W. (1997). Moyamoya disease in adults: Characteristics of clinical presentation and outcome after encephalo-duro-arterio-synangiosis. *Clinical Neurology & Neurosurgery*, *99*(Suppl 2), S151–S155.

Houkin, K., Ishikawa, T., Kuroda, S., & Abe, H. (1998). Vascular reconstruction using interposed small vessels. *Neurosurgery*, *43*(3), 501–505.

Inoue, T. K., Ikezaki, K., Sasazuki, T., Matsushima, T., & Fukui, M. (2000). Linkage analysis of moyamoya disease on chromosome 6. *Journal of Child Neurology*, *15*(3), 179–182.

Kuriyama, S., Kusaka, Y., Fujimura, M., et al. (2008). Prevalence and clinicoepidemiological features of moyamoya disease in Japan: findings from a nationwide epidemiological survey. *Stroke*, *39*(1), 42–47.

Longo, N., Schrijver, I., Vogel, H., et al. (2008). Progressive cerebral vascular degeneration with mitochondrial encephalopathy. *American Journal of Medical Genetics*, *146*(3), 361–367.

Mineharu, Y., Liu, W., Inoue, K., et al. (2008). Autosomal dominant moyamoya disease maps to chromosome 17q25.3. *Neurology*, *70*(24 Pt 2), 2357–2363.

Miyamoto, S., Akiyama, Y., & Nagata, I. (1998). Long-term outcome after STA-MCA anastomosis for moyamoya disease. *Neurosurgical Focus*, *5*, E5.

Scott, R. M., & Smith, E. R. (2009). Epidemiological moyamoya disease and moyamoya syndrome. *New England Journal of Medicine*, *360*, 1226–1237.

Smith, E., & Scott, R. M. (2005). Surgical management of moyamoya syndrome. *Skull Base, 15*, 15–26.

Soriano, S. G., Cowan, D. B., Proctor, M. R., & Scott, R. M. (2002). Levels of soluble adhesion molecules are elevated in the cerebrospinal fluid of children with moyamoya syndrome. *Neurosurgery, 50*(3), 544–549.

Soriano, S. G., Sethna, N. F., & Scott, R. M. (1993). Anesthetic management of children with moyamoya syndrome. *Anesthesia & Analgesia, 77*(5), 1066–1070.

Takagi, Y., Kikuta, K.-I., Sadamasa, N., Nozaki, K., & Hashimoto, N. (2006a). Caspase-3-dependent apoptosis in middle cerebral arteries in patients with moyamoya disease. *Neurosurgery, 59*(4), 894–900.

Takagi, Y., Kikuta, K.-I., Sadamasa, N., Nozaki, K., & Hashimoto, N. (2006b). Proliferative activity through extracellular signal-regulated kinase of smooth muscle cells in vascular walls of cerebral arteriovenous malformations. *Neurosurgery, 58*(4), 740–748; discussion on pp. 740–748.

Uchino, K., Johnston, S. C., Becker, K. J., & Tirschwell, D. L. (2005). Moyamoya disease in Washington State and California. *Neurology, 65*(6), 956–958.

Wakai, K., Tamakoshi, A., Ikezaki, K., et al. (1997). Epidemiological features of moyamoya disease in Japan: findings from a nationwide survey. *Clinical Neurology & Neurosurgery, 99*(Suppl 2), S1–S5.

Binswanger's Disease

11

Sheila A. Alexander

Evidence-Based Nursing Care for Stroke and Neurovascular Conditions,
First Edition. Edited by Sheila A. Alexander.
© 2013 John Wiley & Sons, Inc. Published 2013 by John Wiley & Sons, Inc.

Binswanger's disease, sometimes referred to as subcortical arteriosclerotic encephalopathy, is a small-vessel dementia caused by inadequate blood supply leading to white matter damage and brain atrophy. It is classified as a subcortical dementia because the pathology of the disease is focused on the white matter below the cortical surface. Presence of white matter atrophy is not adequate to diagnose Binswanger's as there are other conditions of white matter atrophy. White matter atrophy in the presence of symptoms of subcortical dementia fully describes Binswanger's disease. The decrease in white matter leads to symptoms related to loss of executive function. Symptoms include memory loss, loss of intellectual function, mood changes, and psychomotor slowing. The loss of function develops over a longer period of time and is progressive in nature if not treated.

Binswanger's is usually diagnosed at 50–60 years old; however, the pathology likely develops over decades before diagnosis. Symptoms progress over an extended period of time with gait disturbances, a later sign, appearing 5 to 10 years after diagnosis. In addition, strokes in small vessels may lead to a sudden increase in symptoms with subsequent stabilization and return to slower progression. While there is minimal literature describing the natural history of Binswanger's disease, these people usually die within 5 years of diagnosis.

PATHOPHYSIOLOGY

Arteriosclerosis causing decreased blood flow to the brain results in generalized brain injury. The arteries of individuals with Binswanger's disease have been damaged over a period of many years due to thickening of the arteries and atherosclerotic plaque development. The vessels lose plasticity and develop a narrow internal lumen. The narrowed lumen and inability to vasodilate to improve cerebral blood flow result in repetitive hypoxic and/or ischemic insults to the brain. In particular the vessels involved are smaller vessels perfusing the subcortical white matter. These vessels arise from the vessels perfusing the basal ganglia, internal capsule, and thalamus (Figure 11.1). Hallmarks of Binswanger's disease include demyelination of axons within the brain, axonal degeneration, and widespread gliosis.

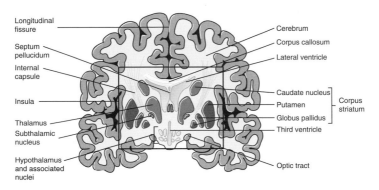

Fig. 11.1 Areas at risk of hypoxia and ischemia in Binswanger's Disease Patients. Reprinted from Tortora, G. J. and Derrickson, B. (2009). *Principles of anatomy and physiology*. Hoboken, NJ: John Wiley & Sons, Inc. with permission.

Disease processes that promote atherosclerosis and arteriosclerosis are risk factors for Binswanger's disease. Increasing age is a non-modifiable risk factor. It is likely that the risk for Binswanger's disease increases with age due to the development of atherosclerosis over the course of a lifetime.

Uncontrolled hypertension is a risk factor for Binswanger's disease. Hypertension increases shear wall stress within blood vessels, initiating inflammation and atherosclerosis development. As the atherosclerotic process progresses, the internal lumen of the blood vessel is decreased. Arterioles also become damaged, leading to a breach in the blood brain barrier.

Uncontrolled or poorly controlled diabetes is a risk factor for Binswanger's disease due to the effects of diabetes on blood vessels. Long-term effects of diabetes, in particular insulin resistance and hyperglycemia, include endothelial cell dysfunction. There is a decrease in nitric oxide synthase production (which helps blood vessels relax), increased endothelin production (which causes vasoconstriction), increased platelet and monocyte adhesion, increased coagulant activity, impaired fibrinolytic activity, and a decrease in fatty acid synthesis induced by lack of insulin and insulin resistance (Sowers, 1998). These changes promote leaky blood vessels and inability to vasodilate normally.

Obstructive sleep apnea is an additional risk factor for Binswanger's disease. In particular obstructive sleep apnea in combination with nocturnal hypertension is frequently seen.

Loss of white matter results in a distinct set of features. Psychomotor slowness – a delay in the time between thinking of and doing a task – is a key feature of Binswanger's disease. Mental manipulation, forgetfulness, and mood/personality changes (irritability, apathy, anxiety, and depression) are classic markers of white matter atrophy, and these symptoms progress with severity of the disease. The slowed mental processing noted in patients with Binswanger's disease leads to impaired concentration, making it difficult to perform everyday tasks. Short-term memory deficits are common, but episodic memory and declarative memory are not affected. Language disorders are a common finding in Binswanger's disease. As the disease progresses, gate changes, movement slowing, and postural changes are common. The gate becomes slow, shuffling, and unsteady. These changes increase risk for falls. Epilepsy, fainting, and loss of bladder control develop later in the disease process. Transient ischemic attacks may occur in Binswanger's disease patients as the intermittent decrease or blockage in blood flow may clear before permanent deficit is formed.

DIAGNOSIS

Initial presentation of Binswanger's disease is often persistent cognitive deficit and/or stroke. Diagnosis is often made with a combination of clinical examination and radioimaging study findings.

Clinical findings suggestive of Binswanger's disease must consider current symptoms, temporal course of development, and medical history. Clinical examination shows a progressive dementia with impaired executive function and normal episodic memory. A gradual progression of symptoms, development of urinary incontinence, and gate changes occurring later are also indicative of Binswanger's disease.

CT scan, magnetic resonance imaging (MRI) and proton MRI spectrography can all be used to determine the hallmark abnormalities in deep brain connectivity seen in Binswanger's disease. Infarction or lesions of central white matter combined with enlarged ventricles are highly suggestive of Binswanger's. Leukoaraiosis is

the term used to describe a decrease in density of white matter commonly seen in Binswanger's disease. The white matter hyperintesities are quite evident around the ventricles and in the diencephalon. Leukoaraiosis occurs in other disease processes, and increases with age, so it is not a definitive diagnosis for Binswanger's disease. Increased leukoaraiosis in multiple areas of the brain is correlated with decreased executive function.

In addition to dementia and radiologic evidence of Binswanger's disease, presence of two of the following may be used:

1. vascular risk factors of evidence of systemic vascular disease;
2. evidence of focal Cerebrovascular disease;
3. evidence of subcortical cerebral dysfunction (Bennett, Wilson, Gilley, & Fox, 1990).

It is important to rule out other causes of dementia in patients with suspected Binswanger's disease. True assessment of the loss of myelination, small infarcts in the deep brain structures, axonal disruption, and microvessel narrowing seen in Binswanger's is best seen on autopsy, so definitive diagnosis is difficult. Genetic testing for CADASIL (see Chapter 8, page 185) or mitochondrial encephalomyopathy, lactic acidosis, and stroke-like episodes (MELAS) may be helpful.

PREVENTION

The most effective method of treating Binswanger's disease is prevention. For patients with a family history of Binswanger's disease, significant atherosclerosis, poorly controlled hypertension, and poorly controlled diabetes, counseling aimed at lifestyle management and treatment adherence should include discussion of risk. Smoking cessation, regular exercise, and a low-fat diet providing proper nutrition and stabilizing blood glucose levels is key to preventing the disease or slowing its progression after diagnosis. While no specific medication has shown superiority in preventing Binswanger disease, the end of goals of maintaining blood pressure within normal limits and blood glucose levels stable should be promoted. Modification of low-density lipoprotein cholesterol with the use of statins and/or antiplatelet medications has been shown to reduce stroke risk and may be beneficial. While this work has

not focused specifically on Binswanger's disease, efforts to limit atherosclerotic progression are likely to slow the progression of the disease process. Management of obstructive sleep apnea is likely to modify disease progression.

SYMPTOM MANAGEMENT

There is no cure for Binswanger's disease. Therapy is aimed at slowing or stopping progression of dementia. Treating the underlying disorder, such as hypertension, has been shown effective in this manner. The majority of treatment for Binswanger's disease is focused on symptom management.

Management of contributing factors

Lifestyle modifications

Patients with Binswanger's disease should be encouraged to lead a more healthful lifestyle upon diagnosis. Smoking cessation, dietary modifications, and regular exercise should be key concepts in counseling. A low-fat diet that provides adequate nutrition and promotes glycemic control should be used to control diabetes and slow progression of atherosclerosis. Exercise has been shown to aid in weight control, blood sugar stabilization, and preventing atherosclerosis.

Blood pressure

Hypertension promotes atherosclerosis and as such is a major causative agent in the pathology related to Binswanger's disease. Controlling blood pressure slows the disease process and therefore symptom progression of the disease. There is minimal empirical evidence suggesting a superior method of hypertension management for slowing Binswanger's pathology.

Diabetes

Diabetes is an additional risk factor for Binswanger's disease development and progression. The vascular changes occurring with uncontrolled diabetes promote atherosclerosis and the decreased cerebral blood flow. Controlling blood sugar slows the disease process, thereby halting or slowing symptom progression of the disease. There is minimal empirical evidence suggesting a superior

method of diabetes management (medications or lifestyle modification). The overall goal is to maintain blood glucose within normal limits.

Cognitive and psychological symptom management

If lifestyle modifications are not adequate to reduce symptom burden, medications should be utilized to treat the underlying condition. Treating the behavioral dysfunction in Binswanger disease frequently employs medications that are useful in other types of dementia.

Memory deficits

Aricept is one drug that has been shown to improve memory deficit in patients with Binswanger disease. Aricept blocks cholinesterase activity, leading to increased acetylcholine in the brain. Memantine is an NMDA glutamate receptor blocker that has been shown to improve cognition and overall functioning and behavior in patients with Binswanger's disease. Nimodipine is a dihydropyridinic calcium antagonist that has been shown to improve cognition in general vascular dementia and subcortical vascular dementia such as Binswanger's disease.

Agitation, aggression, and other behavioral issues

Atypical antipsychotic agents should be used cautiously to treat agitation and other disruptive behaviors. Olanzapine has been shown to decrease agitation, aggression, and violence while not worsening cognition or increasing risk of stroke. Risperidone has similar effects on behavior, but may cause extrapyramidal symptoms or stroke (De Deyn et al., 2005).

Depression and anxiety

Many patients with Binswanger's disease suffer from symptoms of depression and anxiety. Antidepressants are often used to treat symptoms of depression and anxiety. Serotonin-selective reuptake inhibitors, and sertraline and citalopram in particular, have been shown to decrease these symptoms. These medications increase the availability of serotonin in the synapse, promoting neuronal transmission and function. Selective serotonin reuptake inhibitors are helpful for patients with small-vessel dementia and Binswanger's disease, although there have been no randomized clinical trials for this specific population.

REFERENCES

Bennett, D. A., Wilson, R. S., Gilley, D. W., & Fox, J. H. (1990). Clinical diagnosis of Binswanger's disease. *Journal of Neurology, Neurosurgery & Psychiatry*, *53*(11), 961–965.

De Deyn, P. P., Katz, I. R., Brodaty, H., Lyons, B., Greenspan, A., & Burns, A. (2005). Management of agitation, aggression, and psychosis associated with dementia: A pooled analysis including three randomized, placebo-controlled double-blind trials in nursing home residents treated with risperidone. *Clinical Neurology & Neurosurgery*, *107*(6), 497–508.

Sowers, J. R. (1998). Diabetes mellitus and cardiovascular disease in women. *Archives of Internal Medicine*, *158*(6), 617–621.

BIBLIOGRAPHY

Brun, A., Frederiksson, K., & Gustafson, L. (1992). Pure subcortical arteriosclerotic encephalopathy (Binswanger's disease). A clinicopathologic study, II: Pathologic features. *Cerebrovascular Disease*, *2*, 86–92.

Henry, G., Williamson, D., & Tampi, R. R. (2011). Efficacy and tolerability of antidepressants in the treatment of behavioral and psychological symptoms of dementia: A literature review of evidence. *American Journal of Alzheimer's Disease & Other Dementias*, *26*(3), 169–183.

Pantoni, L., del Ser, T., Soglian, A. G., et al. (2005). Efficacy and safety of nimodipine in subcortical vascular dementia: A randomized placebo-controlled trial. *Stroke*, *36*(3), 619–624.

Ramos-Estebanez, C., Moral-Arce, I., Gonzalez-Mandly, A., et al. (2011). Vascular cognitive impairment in small vessel disease: Clinical and neuropsychological features of lacunar state and Binswanger's disease. *Age & Ageing*, *40*(2), 175–180.

Antiphospholipid Syndrome (APS)

12

Alice E. Davis

Evidence-Based Nursing Care for Stroke and Neurovascular Conditions,
First Edition. Edited by Sheila A. Alexander.
© 2013 John Wiley & Sons, Inc. Published 2013 by John Wiley & Sons, Inc.

HISTORICAL PERSPECTIVE

As early as 1906, antiphospholipid antibodies were described as complement-fixing antibodies that reacted with alcoholic extracts of beef heart in syphilis patients. When the essential component within the antigen was identified as cardiolipin, an agglutination test known as Venereal Disease Research Laboratory (VDRL) was developed. Used in screening for syphilis even today, the VDRL has been shown to be transiently or persistently positive even without clinical or serological signs of the disease syphilis. Interestingly, the false positive results were related to nonsyphilitic infections, with persistent positive reactions found in patients with systemic autoimmune diseases, mainly systemic lupus erythematosus (SLE). By 1952, an inhibitor of in vitro coagulation was described in SLE patients by Conley and Hartman (Derksen & de Groot, 2004). The so-called lupus anticoagulant or LA interfered with assemblage of proteins on the phospholipid template, but unlike other inhibitors of coagulation, it did not interfere with bleeding (Derksen, 2004). Later, as a result of false positive VDRLs, complex processing of serum samples, and delays in reporting, immunoassays for detection of cardiolipin (aCL) were developed. Testing for aCL and LC yield overlapping but not identical antibodies as originally presumed. Lastly, in 1990, an autoimmune aCL detected in an ELISA system was found to be directed not at the phospholipids but at phospholipid-binding proteins termed β2 glycoprotein I (β2-GP1). Antibodies causing LA were noted to use β2-GP1, prothrombin, and other plasma proteins as cofactors for lipid binding (Derksen & deGroot, 2004).

In a seminal paper, Hughes (1983) described three unrelated clinical manifestations found commonly in women with SLE. These were recurrent venous thrombosis, central nervous system disease (myelitis, cerebral thrombosis), and recurrent miscarriages. Many of these women also had a common serological abnormality, a circulating aCL responsible for a false positive response to the VDRL test for syphilis. Rates of LA in this group were also higher. At that time, Hughes observed that LA was found in conditions other than SLE and interfered with the binding of phospholipid to form a prothrombin activator, thereby affecting the intrinsic and extrinsic clotting pathways. The paradoxical finding of prolonged partial thromboplastin was associated not with bleeding but with thrombosis.

DEFINING APS

Knowledge generation in APS has been through the contributions of numerous clinical and basic science disciplines including hematology, rheumatology, obstetrics, immunology, neurology, radiology, protein and lipid chemistry, and molecular biology. With advances in understanding of the syndrome, consensus criteria for APS were developed in 1999 (Wilson et al., 1999) and later revised in 2006 (Miyakis et al., 2006) in order to establish a uniform classification system primarily to support rigorous research. Clinicians have now embraced these criteria in order to assist in the differential diagnosis of venous and arterial thrombolic events attributed to APS.

According to the consensus criteria (Miyakis et al., 2006), APS is defined by two major components (Table 12.1). First, there must be at least one antiphospholipid antibody identified in the serum; second, there must be a documented occurrence of at least one of the following clinical features: (1) one or more unexplained thrombotic or thromboembolic events; (2) one or more adverse events related to pregnancy; or (3) unexplained thrombocytopenia or prolongation of a blood coagulation laboratory test (Miyakis et al., 2006). Although not specifically acknowledged as criteria for APS, a vast array of clinical conditions have been associated with APS (Table 12.2). Clinical suspicion for APS may be heightened if any one or combinations of these clinical conditions occur.

TYPES

There are three distinct types of APS identified in the literature. The term primary has been assigned to APS occurring in the absence of any other related diseases. APS has also been identified in the setting of an underlying disease especially other autoimmune conditions such as systemic lupus erythematosus (SLE). If APS coexists with other diseases, it is considered secondary APS. Catastrophic APS has been described in patients who develop severe life-threatening disease. Although rare, catastrophic APS is diagnosed if there is manifestation of the disease in three or more organs over a period of one week; there is histologic confirmation of thrombosis; and laboratory confirmation of antiphospholipid antibodies. Even with aggressive therapy, mortality for catastrophic APS approaches 50% (Asherson et al, 2003).

Table 12.1 Summary of revised consensus criteria for antiphospholipid syndrome

APS present if at least one clinical and one laboratory criteria below are met

Clinical Criteria	
Vascular Thrombosis	Arterial, venous, or small-vessel thrombosis in any tissue or organ (one or more clinical episodes confirmed by objective validated criteria (imaging or histopathology confirmation
Pregnancy Mortality	One or more unexplained fetal deaths at or beyond 10 weeks gestation (normal fetal documented by ultrasound or direct fetal examination)
	One or more premature births (before 34 weeks) of morphologically normal neonate due to eclampsia or severe pre-eclampsia or recognized placental insufficiency
	Three unexplained consecutive spontaneous abortions before the 10th week of gestation, excluding those related to maternal, hormonal, or chromosomal abnormalities
Laboratory Criteria	
	Lupus anticoagulant (LA) present in plasma on two or more occasions 12 weeks apart (must follow specific detection guideline criteria)
	Anticardiolipin (aCL) antibody of IgG and/or IgM isotype in serum plasma (medium to high titer) on two or more occasions 12 weeks apart (standard ELISA)
	Anti β_2 glycoprotein antibody of IgG and/or IgM (titer 99th percentile standard ELISA) on two or more occasions 12 weeks apart.

Adapted from: Miyakis, S., Lockshin, M. D., Atsumi, T., Branch, D.W., Brey, R.L., et al. (2006). International consensus statement on an update of the classification criteria for definite antiphospholipid syndrome (APS). *Journal of Thrombosis and Haemostasis, 4*, 295–306.

While there has been continued recognition and acceptance of the clinical and laboratory features of APS established by the consensus conferences, numerous variants thought to be microvascular or microangiopathic precursors are being described. This microangiopathic antiphospholipid syndrome (MAPS) has several but not all the features described in the APS criteria. However, there is suspicion that this subset of disorders such as livedo reticularis, choreas of the nervous system, heart valve lesions, thrombocytopenia, and other clinical conditions are often followed for years and are later diagnosed as APS (Asherson, 2006). Thus, there is growing

Table 12.2 Systemic complications identified with APS

System	Manifestation
General	Behçet's disease (vasculitis), fatigue, aches and pains
Venous	Deep venous thrombosis
Arterial	Organ thrombosis, limb pain
Pregnancy	Miscarriages, early and late pregnancy losses, infertility, intrauterine growth retardation, eclampsia
Brain	Headache, migraines, cerebral ischemia (stroke, TIA), memory loss, movement and balance disorders (chorea), transverse myelopathy, myelitis, seizures, atypical multiple sclerosis (MS)
Heart	Myocardial infarction, valve disease, murmurs, angina
Lungs	Pulmonary embolism, pulmonary hypertension
Kidney	Hypertension, microangiographic nephropathy, arterial and renal vein thrombosis, proteinuria, adrenal infarction and hemorrhage
Liver	Portal hypertension, Budd-Chiari Syndrome (obstruction of hepatic venous outflow), thrombosis
Gastrointestinal	Ischemic bowel, abdominal pain, hematochezia
Blood	Hemolytic anemia, thrombocytopenia
Ocular/Eyes	Amaurosis, retinal thrombosis, visual loss due to clots, visual field loss, Sjogren's syndrome
Skin	Livedo reticularis, Raynouds
Musculoskeletal	Avascular necrosis of bone
MS-like features	Numbness and tingling, double vision, visual field loss, motor weakness

support for recognition and aggressive treatment of persons presenting with thrombotic microangiopathy and laboratory evidence of antiphospholipid antibodies who share common but not identical predisposing factors including infection and drug exposure and who exhibit clinical and hematological signs (thrombocytopenia and hemolytic anemia) of APS (Asherson, 2006; Asherson & Cervera, 2007).

PATHOGENESIS
The exact mechanism responsible for the dysregulation of blood coagulation and resulting thrombosis is not clear. Exposure to an infectious agent in susceptible persons is one commonly accepted

explanation. However, with the exception of the many rheumatic diseases, specifically SLE, the underlying cause of such suscepti-bilities is unknown. Several mechanisms have been postulated to explain the molecular basis of the prothrombic process associated with the antibodies. Antiphospholipid antibodies are thought to (1) bind and activate endothelial cells inducing expression of adhesion molecules and tissue factor; (2) interfere with endogenous anticoag-ulation mechanisms (annexin V binding to anionic phospholipids); (3) interfere with fibrinolysis; (4) inhibit protein C pathways with inhibition of antithrombin; (5) activate the complement cascade; and (6) bind and activate platelets (Ortel, 2005; Belilos & Carson, 2009). There is growing support for an inflammatory etiology in APS, especially in pregnancy. Activation of complement is thought to be responsible for inflammatory mediated tissue damage to the placenta (Girardi, Lockshin, & Salamon, 2007).

There is some support for a "second-hit" theory as a basis for development of APS – that is, once aPL are present, development of the full-blown syndrome occurs. Numerous clinical conditions are thought to be potential delivery mechanisms in the "second-hit" theory and include: cigarette smoking, immobilization, pregnancy, post-partum period, use of oral contraceptives, hormone replace-ment therapy, malignancy, nephrotic syndrome, hypertension, and hyperlipidemia (Erkan & Lockshin, 2004).

PREVALENCE

Presence of aPL has been found in a cross-section of individuals and age groups. Reports from a study conducted by Cervera, Piette, Khamashta, Shoenfeld, and Camps (2002) addressed the clinical and immunological manifestations and patterns of disease expres-sion. In a cohort of 1,000 patients (820 female and 180 male), mean age of 42 +/− 14 years, "primary" APS was found in 53.1% of patients and was associated with SLE (secondary) in 36.2%, lupus-like syndrome in 5.0%, or with other diseases in 5.9%.

There is no defined race predominance. A higher occurrence in females has been linked with secondary APS that is consistent with prevalence of SLE and other connective tissues disease in women. In healthy persons, aPL is generally transient, but persistence may indicate susceptibility of APS. SLE is the most common condition of the rheumatic disease with aPL presence (LA, aCL, β2-GP1), but aPL (LA and aCL) has also been found in scleroderma and psoriatic arthritis. Bacterial, viral, and parasitic infections have been associated with the presence of aPL, especially aCL (IgM isotype), with occasional occurrence of thrombotic events, but these conditions are not usually associated with anti-ß2-GP-I activity. Certain medications have also been connected to aPL activity, especially of the IgM isotype. Although rarely associated with thrombosis, the medications identified are phenothiazines, phenytoin, hydralazine, procainamide, quinidine, ethosuximide, alpha interferon, amoxicillin, chlorothiazide, oral contraceptives, and propranolol (Merrill, Shen, Gugnani, Lahita, & Mongey, 1997; Belilos & Carsons, 2009). Other conditions where aPL have been identified are solid organ tumors and hematologic malignancies and other generalized chronic conditions such as immune thrombocytopenia, sickle cell anemia, pernicious anemia, diabetes mellitus, inflammatory bowel disease, dialysis, and Klinefelter syndrome (Cervera & Asherson 2003; Bermas, Erkan, & Schur, 2010).

LABORATORY TESTING

In addition to clinical manifestations, the diagnosis of APS depends on laboratory detection of aPL, specifically lupus anticoagulant (LA), anticardiolipin antibody (aCL), and anti-ß2 glycoprotein-I. For diagnosing APS, testing for aPL on two or more occasions at least 12 weeks apart and no more than 5 years prior to demonstration of clinical signs is recommended (Bermas, Erkan, & Schur, 2010). Specific aPL and interpretation of findings are presented in Table 12.3. Testing for the presence of multiple aPL and repeat testing over time aid in the exclusion of patients with transitory reactivity. There is some concern for a seronegative APS class of patients – that is, patients with strong clinical indicators for APS but where laboratory support for the syndrome is lacking (Hughes & Khamashta, 2003). A review of the specific aPL, the anticipated results, and testing recommendations are reviewed in more detail below.

Lupus Anticoagulant (LA) is a misnomer; it is not a diagnostic test for SLE. Rather it was named for a group of phospholipid inhibitors related to thrombolic complications. The association between thrombotic events and antiphospholipid activity was initially described in SLE patients, hence the name LA (Hughes,

Table 12.3 Interpretation of laboratory studies for APS

aPL or Factor Type	Testing Method	Results	Evaluation
Lupus Anticoagulant Panel (LA)	aPTT dRVVT KCT dPT	Need two or more tests for accurate screening	Very sensitive: false (−) results if platelets not adequately removed; false (+) if heparin is present (Derkson)
Cardiolipin Antibodies (aCL) IgG IgM IgA (Renan)	ELISA Assay	Medium or high titer >40GPL or MPL, or >99th percentile for the testing laboratory. IgA (use if APS suspected but other aPL tests are negative)	Seen in autoimmune disorders (SLE), acute Infections, HIV/AIDS, cancer, some drug classes
$\beta 2$ glycoprotein-1 (β2-GP1).	ELISA Assay	Antibodies to ß2-glycoprotein-I (ß2-GP-I) of IgG or IgM isotype	Very specific for APS but alone is less sensitive than LA and aCL combined
Thrombocytopenia	Platelet Count	Platelet count <50–150 micro	Usually moderate thrombocytopenia in APS

dRVVT = dilute Russell viper venom time
dAPTT = dilute activated partial thromboplastin time
KCT = kaolin clotting time
dPT = dilute prothrombin time
Created from information found in Rouby (1994); Derkson & de Groot (2004); Bermas et al. (2010); Koniari et al. (2010).

1983). LA is a panel of sequential tests that depend on phospholipid reagents (Table 12.3). An LA panel should be initiated when a prolongation of the prothrombin time is noted in a patient not receiving anticoagulants or unfractionated heparin. LA prolongs the clotting time of phospholipid-dependent coagulation tests (such as protime). Similarly, false positive results can be encountered with patients on anticoagulants as clotting times will be prolonged. Thus, ideal testing would occur when all antithrombotic agents have been discontinued (Derkson & de Groot, 2004; Lim, 2009). LA is considered highly sensitive but not specific for thromboembolic risk in APS patients. A battery of laboratory tests should follow an initial prolonged clotting study and include dRVVT, dAPTT, KCT, and dPT. LA is present if any of the tests are positive but two or more positive results provide stronger support for APS. Adherence to the published international guidelines for testing LA is recommended (Derksen & de Groot, 2004; Koniari et al., 2010).

Cardiolipin is a major component of the inner membrane of the mitochondria, necessary for energy production and found in the heart muscle. Using the enzyme-linked immunosorbent assays (ELISAs), three isotopes of aCL directed against cardiolipin have been identified: IgG, IgM, and IgA. A limitation to the test is the presence of anti 2 glycoprotein I, a co-factor determined to be necessary for the reaction between aCL antibodies and phospholipid binding proteins. Such a reaction, even if a small, results in a positive result (see below). Therefore, in evaluating IgG and/or IgM test results, only moderate or high titers (>40 units GPL or MPL or >99th percentile for the testing laboratory) should be considered positive for aCL (Pengo et al., 2009). Although a positive aCL should only be considered in the differential diagnosis of APS, there is strong evidence linking aCL with thrombosis, especially in SLE. Moreover, aCL is more useful than LA in patients undergoing immunosuppressive therapy. Lower titers have been associated with false positive results yielding only a small percentage of positive results when repeat studies are conducted. Laboratory results should always be evaluated based on clinical findings before the diagnosis of APS is made. Repeat testing is recommended as transiently increased aCL may occur in the setting of viral or other infections. A confirmatory aCL, anti-ß2-GP-I, or LA test obtained at least 12 weeks after the initial positive test increases confidence in the diagnosis (Burmas & Schur, 2010).

LA and aCL antibodies do not react with phospholipids themselves but with phospholipid-binding plasma proteins (cofactors). The established co-factors are anti-β2 glycoprotein I for ELISA and anti 2 glycoprotein I and prothrombin for antibodies causing LA (Roubey, 1994). This explains earlier notions that aCL and LC refer to related, but not necessarily similar, antibodies. To classify a patient as having APS, both aCL and LA assays have to be performed.

False negative tests — Some patients with clinical features consistent with APS do not have detectable aCL, anti-ß2-GP-I antibodies, or a positive LA test, especially at the time of thrombosis. Other aPL tests that can be considered in this setting are those directed against phosphatidylserine, phosphatidylinositol, and prothrombin (Bertolaccini et al., 2005; Giannakopoulos, Passam, Ioannou, & Krilis, 2009). However, little is known about the sensitivity, specificity, and clinical significance of testing for these antibodies. Thus, if the initial aPL tests (aCL, anti-ß2-GP-I, LA test) are negative, screening for inheritable and acquired disorders of coagulation (e.g., clotting factor deficiencies) should be strongly considered before ordering additional aPL tests (Bermas et al., 2010).

As described above, there are numerous pitfalls in the laboratory detection of aPL due to the lack of standardized guidelines for screening. Obviously, a non-uniform classification of patients as positive or negative for aPL hinders comparison of results from different clinical studies and contributes to discrepant findings for associations between aPL and pregnancy outcome, as well as to the wide variation in reported frequencies of aPL in different populations (Derkson & de Groot, 2004).

CLINICAL MANIFESTATIONS

Clinical manifestations of APS, especially thrombotic manifestations, are far-reaching and involve almost every system in the body. As seen in Table 12.1, there is a vast array of systems and conditions associated with APS. Cervera et al. (2002) reported those patients with secondary APS (associated with SLE) had more episodes, and *livedo reticularis* occurred more often in females. In males, there was a higher rate of epilepsy, myocardial infraction, and arterial thrombosis, especially in the lower legs and feet. Moreover, men who were diagnoses with APS after age 50 and had a higher frequency of stroke and angina. In the younger cohort (onset of disease before age 15), there were more episodes of chorea and jugular vein thrombosis.

Because there is such a vast array of clinical features associated with APS, the following section addresses the most prevalent and most well documented of the thrombotic conditions. These include the clinical manifestations associated with pregnancy, cardiovascular and nervous systems, and bleeding clotting abnormalities.

Thrombosis in pregnancy

The presence of aPL has been associated with early pregnancy losses as well as fetal death in advanced pregnancy. Numerous studies have identified aPL as causative for pregnancy-related morbidities in patients with SLE healthy nulliparous women (Hughes, 1983; Lynch et al., 1994). Women with three or more consecutive miscarriages who persistently test positive for aPL have up to 90% chance of fetal loss if not treated for APS. In one study, intrauterine fetal deaths (Out, Kooijman, Bruinse, & Derksen, 1991) were highly associated with placental thrombosis and infarction. Clinical complications including pre-eclampsia, intrauterine growth restriction, fetal distress, and premature delivery also rose in women with aPL (Branch, Silver, Blackwell, Reading, & Scott, 1992; Lima, Khamashta, Buchanan, Kerslake, Hunt, & Hughes, 1996). Risk factors for thrombosis are also a concern during early pregnancy; therefore, knowledge of previous thrombolic events and identification of current organ damage must be obtained. Complications such as severe pre-eclampsia or eclampsia, elevated liver enzymes, or low platelet counts (HELLP syndrome) may accelerate APS pathology and necessitate pregnancy termination. It is known that thrombogenesis occurs not only during pregnancy but also during the postpartum period (Bates, Greer, Pabinger, Sofaer, & Hirsh, 2008). Continually monitoring for pre-eclampsia and HELLP syndrome is important. Ischemic stroke has been reported as a common thrombotic manifestation weeks into the postpartum period. Special concern should be given to the SLE pregnant women who are at high risk for maternal complications following delivery but who also has risk for maternal and fetal complications before delivery (Girardi et al., 2007).

Although fetal complications and death are reported in APS and SLE pregnancies, they are rarely caused by thrombolic events. Rather, fetal death has been associated with reduction of amniotic fluid, placental insufficiency, small placental size, restricted fetal growth, and starvation. Pathology reports of placentas have demonstrated increased levels of aPL, specifically IgG and β_2GPI, along with a variety of vascular and inflammatory changes (Girardi et al., 2007).

Thrombosis of the cardiovascular system

APS seems to have widespread consequences to the heart and cardiovascular system. Coronary artery disease (CAD), valvular heart disease, dilated cardiomyopathy, pulmonary hypertension, and intracardiac thrombus have been reported (Hedge et al., 2007; Weiss et al., 2008). Arthrosclerosis appears to be accelerated in APS patients, and risk factors are inflammatory and immuopathologic as opposed to the lifestyle and hereditary factors demonstrated in classic CAD (Weiss et al., 2008). There are several noteworthy features related to valvular disease: (1) mitral valve affected more commonly than aortic and tricuspid; (2) valve leaflet thickening is due to immune complexes; and (3) presence of thrombotic, fibrotic, calcified lesions (Gorki, Malinovski, & Stanbridge, 2008). Because of the close association between APS and SLE, SLE can also cause valve disease. Valve replacement is patient specific and based on age of onset and need for long-term anticoagulation. Thrombotic risk is pervasive encompassing pulmonary and systemic emboli involving the right-sided heart chambers most frequently. Venous and arterial thrombosis of the lower extremities is also prevalent with a tendency toward repetitive (same type) but sporadic episodes despite persistent presence of aPL over long periods of time. The sporadic nature of large thrombolic events in the presence of aPL has lead to speculation that thrombosis is occurring in smaller vessels (microvascular), contributing to organ damage and later organ dysfunction. Targeted organs and vessels are kidneys, brain, and heart vasculature (Konairi et al., 2010). The abnormalities associated with bleeding are found in the thrombocytopenia section discussed below.

Thrombosis of the nervous system

Nervous system findings associated with APS have been identified as transient ischemic attacks, cerebral infarct (thrombolic or embolic), cerebral venous thrombosis, headaches, migraines, visual disturbances, mononeuritis multiplex, seizures, and myelitis (Levine, Deegan, Futrell, & Welch, 1990; Cervera et al., 2002; Hawkins, Gatenby, Tuck, Danta, & Andrews, 2006). These nervous system disorders have been identified in persons as young as 15 years of age (Hawkins et al., 2006).

Controversial results regarding stroke treatment and recurrent thromboembolic events were reported in the Antiphospholipid Antibodies and Stroke Study (APASS) (Levine et al., 2004). APASS, a large, randomized, double-blind trial, was an arm of the Warfarin vs. Aspirin Recurrent Stroke Study (WARSS). The APASS study sought to identify association between the presence of aPL at the time of an initial ischemic stroke and subsequent thromboembolic events (Levine et al., 2004). When compared to patients without aPL present at the time of stroke, patients with aPL did not have an increased risk for recurrent thromboembolic events, nor were treatment outcomes using warfarin or aspirin different from non-aPL patients.

Thrombocytopenia

Despite the prothrombic features of APS, thrombocytopenia, defined as a platelet count <50–150 microL, is a frequent finding, occurring in 20% of APS patients and 40% in patient with secondary APS associated with SLE (Lim, 2009). Thrombocytopenia was found more commonly associated with LA (55%) and aCL (29%). Moreover, in patients with thrombocytopenia associated with autoimmune disorders, aPL were frequently present. This was demonstrated in 70–80 % of patients with SLE and 30–40% with idiopathic (ITP) thrombocytopenia purpura. (McNeil, Chesterman, & Krillis, 1991; Cervera et al., 2002).

Several theories as to the etiology of the thrombocytopenia have been offered. One theory suggests an occurrence of an immune-mediated clearance of platelets. Another proposes that aPL interact with platelets in such a way as to trigger platelet aggregation and thrombosis. There is support for this theory in both in vitro and in vivo studies where aPL binds with platelets and increases platelet aggregation and activation (Campbell, Pierangeli, Wellhausen, & Harris, 1995). This also supports the frequent concomitant findings of thrombotic complications in the setting of thrombocytopenia in these patients. It has been noted that despite the thrombocytopenia, APS is not typically associated with bleeding complications (Cuadrado, Mujic, Monoz, Khamashta, & Hughes, 1997; Finazzi, 1997; Lim, 2009).

Generalized APS

"Catastrophic" is the term used to define an accelerated and destructive form of APS resulting in multiorgan failure. This life-threatening form of APS, also known as Asherson's syndrome, may be precipitated by infection, lupus flare, or malignancy and requires astute clinical awareness, aggressive therapy, and close monitoring.

Although only 1% of APS patients experience catastrophic APS, preliminary classification criteria were developed (Asherson et al., 2003).

Three clear aims for the optimal management of catastrophic APS are suggested: (1) treat any precipitating factors including timely use of antibiotics if for suspected infection, surgical removal of any suspected necrotic organs, and precautions in patients with APS who require surgical or invasive procedures; (2) prevent or treat potential or ongoing thrombotic events and suppress activation of cytokines to avert a cytokine "storm"; and (3) institute anticoagulation therapy. Commonly used treatments for catastrophic APS include intravenous heparin followed by oral anticoagulants, corticosteroids, or immunosuppressive therapy (plasmapheresis and intravenous gamma globulins) and, if associated with lupus flare, cyclophosphamide (Asherson et al., 2003).

APPROACH TO DIAGNOSIS
History
High index of suspicion should trigger a thorough history and review of systems. For example, obstetric history, arterial or venous thrombosis before age 45, or unusual site for arterial and venous thrombosis should activate further inquiry. The history should focus on the type and frequency of thromboembolic events, adverse pregnancy outcomes, unexplained prolongation of coagulant tests, hemolytic anemias, thrombocytopenia, history of heart murmurs, cardiac valve vegetation, thrombosis risk factors, medications known to be associated with aPL production (phenothiazines, hydralazine, procainamide, and phenytoin), and associated illness, especially SLE (see Table 12.2) (Ortel, 2005; Belilos & Carson, 2009).

Physical examination
Abnormal findings of physical examination are primarily associated with ischemia to the skin, viscera, or nervous system. These may include presence of livedo reticularis, deep venous thrombosis (DVT), peripheral edema and leg swelling, digital ischemia, gangrene, leg ulcers, splinter hemorrhages, ascites, or neurological signs and symptoms consistent with a stroke.

Diagnostic testing

Laboratory Tests — The section on laboratory testing above provides precise detail on specific aPL laboratory tests. Consideration for testing should be given to individuals whose history generates a high index of suspicion and those with: (1) a new, unexplained, spontaneous venous or arterial thromboembolic event; (2) an atypical thromboembolic or unusual presentation of a thromboembolic event; (3) a history or pregnancy mortality; or (4) unexplained thrombocytopenia or bleeding disorder (Ortel, 2005; Belilos & Carson, 2009).

A complete blood cell count (CBC) should be analyzed for evidence of thrombocytopenia or hemolytic anemia. Additional laboratory testing should include prothrombin time, partial thromboplastin time, and serology for syphilis.

Imaging studies

Diagnostic imaging studies should include confirmation of a thrombotic event involving the brain (stroke), chest (pulmonary embolism), or abdomen using computerized tomography (CT) scan or magnetic resonance imaging (MRI). Doppler ultrasound studies should be used to detect deep venous thrombosis (DVT) and echocardiograms used for inspection of the heart and cardiac valves (Belilos & Carson, 2009).

TREATMENT

Once aPL have been identified or APS has been diagnosed, several approaches to care have been recommended. Patients with known or suspected APS can be evaluated in the outpatient setting unless a significant clinical event occurs that warrants hospitalization. There is no strong evidence to treat positive aPL patients who are asymptomatic unless they demonstrate high risk factors for an initial thrombotic event (Ruffatti et al., 2011). Outpatient care should include monitoring for any clinical events, management of potential thrombotic risk factors (hypertension, hypercholesterolemia, elevated homocysteine levels,) management of medications doses if undergoing anticoagulant therapy (Table 12.4), and monitoring laboratory values such as PT/INR. Education must be an integral

Table 12.4 Commonly used medications in APS

Drug	Classification	Mechanism of Action	Dose	Indications
Aspirin	Antiplatelet	Exact action unknown, inhibits platelet aggregation	81 mg PO	Used in pregnancy w/o hx of thrombosis, stroke
Clopidogrel	Antiplatelet			
Heparin	Anticoagulant	Binds to antithrombin III, causing inactivation of thrombin and other factors	5–10,000 Units SQ q12 hrs 1–2,000 Units IV per protocol	IV infusion to warfarin conversion (Thrombotic events); Prophylaxis during pregnancy or until warfarin therapeutic
Prednisone	Corticosteroid	Unknown; inhibits multiple inflammatory cytokines providing corticosteroid effects	Individualized dosing	Used in nonthrombotic autoimmune disorders such as thrombocytopenia
Warfarin (Coumadin)	Anticoagulant	Inhibits hepatic synthesis of vitamin K dependent coagulation factors	2–5 mg PO until target PT/INR achieved or may be increased in high-risk patients	Long-term use for recurrent thrombotic events
Hydroxychloroquine (plaquenil)	Antimalarial; antirheumatic	Inhibits nucleic acid and acute phase responses of rheumatoid factor and other enzymes	6–7 mg/kg/d single or divided doses	Used in prophylactic therapy due to its antithrombotic properties
Cyclophosphamide (Rituximab)	Immunosuppressive	Chimeric anti CD-20 monoclonal antibody interferes w DNA replication	0.5–1 g/m IVPB or 2–3 mg/kg/d PO	Used in CAPS refractory and APS
Immunoglobulin (IV route)	Immunoglobulin	Unknown; reestablishes normal immunoregulatory pathways		Used in CAPS; may prevent late pregnancy complications

part of outpatient management, with emphasis on early recognition of a clinical event, smoking cessation, avoidance of oral contraception and estrogen replacement therapies, preventing long-term immobilization, and stressing the importance of pregnancy planning (Belilos & Carson, 2009). Special concern should be given to patients who are preparing for surgery and who are withdrawing from anticoagulants such as warfarin; post-operative patients, especially if the patient is in a hypercoagulable state; and patients diagnosed with known APS or SLE. Even in mild cases, thrombosis can be triggered by surgery, infection, or mild anticoagulation.

To assure the safest outcomes for hospitalized patients, a multidisciplinary management approach must be taken. This includes consults to neurology, rheumatology, hematology, and obstetrics (during pregnant); services of a cardiologist, pulmonologist, hepatologist, and ophthomologist may be needed depending on clinical manifestations. Nursing care includes astute serial assessments and monitoring for DVTs, skin eruptions, cerebral vascular events, or cardiac events. Precise titration of heparin drips for anticoagulation, maintaining PTT within therapeutic range, analyzing PT/INR results in early phase diagnoses and once oral anticoagulation therapy is initiated, and continued evaluation of other tests of anticoagulation, including those for anemia, are warranted.

Whether outpatient or inpatient, treatment is determined by the individual needs of a patient. Treatment tiers include primary and secondary prophylaxis, treatment geared to specific clinical manifestations, or preoperative preparation for a surgical procedure (Table 12.5). Clinical manifestations or conditions requiring treatment include venous and arterial sources of thrombosis, pre and post partum pregnancy care, thrombocytopenia, cerebrovascular or cardiac events, and patients being consideration for surgery. Antithrombotic therapy is the mainstay of treatment with medications such as heparin, warfarin, and aspirin being used most frequently (Table 12.4).

Primary prophylaxis has been suggested in asymptomatic patients who may demonstrate risk factors for an initial thrombotic event. Patients with hypertension and or medium to high titers of IgG aCL have been identified as asymptomatic carriers who may benefit from thromboprophylaxis if faced with a high-risk event (Ruffatti et al., 2011).

Table 12.5 APS treatment recommendations by clinical manifestation

Clinical Manifestation	Suggested Therapy
Pregnancy morbidity (Girardi et al., 2007; Bates et al., 2008; Belilos & Carsons, 2009; Lim, 2009)	Goal to prevent further therapy losses rather than treat thrombosis. Low-dose ASA w prophylactic or intermediate-dose unfractionated heparin or prophylactic LMWH w/o hx of thrombosis. Discontinue warfarin before pregnancy due to its teratogenic effects (abnormal development). Treat three months post-partum during partum.
DVT (Belilos & Carsons, 2009; Lim, 2009)	Initial: Heparin, LMWH 4-5 days w warfarin overlap, in high risk for bleeding or thrombocytopenia use unfractionated heparin
	Long term: Warfarin or Vit K antagonists keep INR 2-3; continuous monitoring of INR/ Hgb in presence of thrombocytopenia, some support for adding aspirin to anticoagulation regimen.
Stroke (arterial thromboembolism) (Derksen et al., 2003; Albers et al., 2008; Lim, 2009).	APASS study recommendations: ASA or warfarin for first-time stroke but therapy controversial since no patients in the study meet APS criteria. Anticoagulation not contraindicated in thrombocytopenia but close monitoring for bleeding is important.
Cardiac (arterial thromboembolism) (Hirsh et al., 2008)	MI: Placed on long-term warfarin to achieve INR 2.0-3.0, but there is no data to support the treatment recommendations
	Peripheral arterial thromboembolism: Same treatment as DVT but duration of treatment is not addressed; continuous monitoring of patient risk factors is necessary.
Inflammation (Girardi et al., 2007)	Inflammation identified in models of APS and pregnancy. Heparin has been demonstrated to have anticomplement effects, and may limit antibody targeting of trophoblasts, thus decreasing aPL-mediated damage.
Thrombocytopenia (Lim, 2009)	If APS-associated thrombocytopenia, then treatment similar to that used w ITP is started including steroids, IVIG, immunosuppressive agents, rituximab. Treatment initiated to minimize bleeding or antithrombotic events. No trials reported for treatment, but recommendations suggest treat if there is overt bleeding or when bleeding risk outweighs treatment risk; OK to treat when platelets are 20–30,000 according to ITP consensus guidelines. Pregnant women may require treatment to achieve homeostasis at delivery or for epidural catheter placement.
APS and bleeding (Lim, 2009)	Less often a complication compared to thrombosis in APS. If bleeding occurs, determine source, stop antithrombotic agents, administer reversal medications (protamine sulfate for heparin and Vit K for warfarin, consider transfusions of RBCs, FFP, and platelets as needed). Simultaneous bleeding and thrombosis require management of most life-threatening problem. If high index for bleeding, hold anticoagulants.
Cardiac surgery (Koniari et al., 2010)	Start unfractionated heparin before coronary bypass surgery; monitoring activated clotting time may be problematic since it is phospholipid dependent; if MWH used no need for monitoring.
CAPS (Belilos & Carsons, 2009)	Plasmapheresis, w/wo IV IG, steroids.

A high incidence of reoccurrence has been documented in patients who have had an initial thromboembolic episode, placing them at higher risk for future events. According to Pengo et al. (2009) patients who tested positive for three aPL tests were at highest risk for reoccurrence. The type of initial episode (arterial, venous, or pregnancy) was not predictive of the type of reoccurrence. Since all patients had similar incidences of reoccurring thromboembolic events, the aPL profile, not the clinical manifestation, more closely predicted reoccurrence. This high incidence of reoccurrence emphasizes the need for long-term antithrombotic therapy (Pengo, 2009). There is, however, considerable debate related to the treatment of these patients using anticoagulation, understanding the necessity to balance prevention of further events with prevention of major hemorrhagic complications.

There is also continued debate on the type and extent of treatment as well as prophylactic treatment recommendations for specific types of clinical manifestations. While there has been considerable investigation on the proper management of APS, reported studies lack agreement due to differences in study design, methods, variability in admission criteria, and other methodological issues (Ruiz-Irastorza & Khamashta, 2005).

There is support to treat first-time venous thromboembolic events with anticoagulation (Lim, 2009), and the optimal target INR for patients with aPL and thromboembolism has been examined by numerous investigators (Buller et al., 2004; Hirsh, Guyatt, Albers, Harrington, & Schünemann, 2008) (Table 12.4). In the studies conducted by Crowther and Wisloff (2005), Finazzi et al. (2005), and Pengo et al. (2010), lowest risk for reoccurrence of thromboembolic events was on warfarin therapy with target INR range between 2 and 3. Higher INR ranges were deemed unnecessary and were associated with adverse bleeding events in several trials (Crowther & Wisloff, 2005; Finazzi et al., 2005), but antiplatelet therapy with aspirin was insufficient to prevent recurrent thromboembolic events in these patients. The optimal treatment for patients with arterial thromboembolic events remains controversial, but Pengo et al. (2010) reported less arterial thromboembolic events with anticoagulation therapy suggesting this subgroup could also benefit from long-term anticoagulation therapy. The addition of low-dose aspirin is an option. Alternative treatment modalities still under investigation include use of low molecular weight heparin (Pengo et al., 2009), hematopoietic stem cell transplant, or methods that lower aPL titer such as rituximab and plasmapheresis (Tsagalis, Psimenou, Nakopoulou, & Laggouranis, 2010) (Table 12.4).

Numerous investigations have addressed treatment issues related to APS and stroke. The use of aspirin following stroke has been recommended (Derksen, de Groot, & Kappelle, 2003; Pengo et al., 2009). The Stroke Prevention in Reversible Ischemia Trial (SPIRIT) (1997) was an effort to determine the efficacy and safety between low-dose aspirin and anticoagulant drugs. Reported results documented excessive deaths from vascular origins in the higher-intensity anticoagulation group, and the trial was stopped early. Recommendations were not given for lower-level ranges of anticoagulation. In the controversial APASS study (Levine et al., 2004), stroke patients did not demonstrate an increased risk for thromboembolic events, and treatment outcomes were not different between warfarin and aspirin. Ruiz-Isarstorza & Khamashta (2005) advocated that therapy following stroke in the presence of APS must address the individual needs of the patient, the severity of the initial stroke, concomitant vascular risk factors, potential for future thrombotic events, bleeding history, and age. In fact, they supported the use of oral anticoagulation at elevated ranges in high-risk patients. More recent recommendations from the American College of Chest Physicians (Albers, Schunemann, Easton, Sacco, & Teal, 2008) promote the use of antiplatelet agents over oral anticoagulation in transient ischemic attacks or non-cardioembolic stroke.

Keeping in mind the controversies and pitfalls of the current state of treatment in APS, Ortel (2005) has developed a simple rubric for clinical treatment, which emphasizes a high index of suspicion based on event history, understanding of laboratory values, and evidence-based treatment of the clinical event.

Step 1: Identify the background for the clinical event: (1) new, spontaneous venous thromboembolic event, (2) young patient, new arterial thromboembolic event, (3) atypical thromboembolic event, or (4) unusual presentations of a thromboembolic event

Step 2: Confirm baseline protime (PT) is normal, or if abnormal, confirm presence of aPL with further laboratory studies (see Table 12.3).

Step 3: Treatment – venous: (1) oral anticoagulation INR range between 2 and 3; (2) identify and treat co-morbid prothrombic states such as homocysteine with folic acid; (3) for recurrent events, manage INR at a higher range, use an alternate anticoagulant such as low molecular weight heparin, or initiate immunomodulartory therapies. Treatment – arterial; (1) higher INR ranges than venous recommendations (are controversial); (2) identify and treat co-morbid prothrombic states such as elevated cholesterol or hypertension; (3) recurrent events same as venous event treatment.

SUMMARY

To date, the research evidence provides direction for the recognition of APS through laboratory and clinical manifestations and provides guidelines for prophylactic and thromboembolic treatment. Consensus guidelines suggest clinical suspicion for APS should be heightened if one of the following occurs: (1) one or more unexplained thrombotic or thromboembolic events; (2) one or more adverse events related to pregnancy; or (3) unexplained thrombocytopenia or prolongation of a blood coagulation laboratory test (Miyakis et al., 2006). Investigations continue to be under way regarding optimal therapy for all APS-related thromboembolic risk or events. Oral anticoagulation may be safe and efficacious in some situations and may be insufficient in other areas. The risk of bleeding from heighted anticoagulation coupled with the complications of thrombocytopenia requires alternate strategies for high-risk groups. And there has been little information shed on the use of alternate therapies, prognostic indicators, or long-term outcomes for this group of patients.

REFERENCES

Aguilar-Valenzuela, R., Seif, A., Alarcon, G., et al. (2009). Isolated elevated levels of IgA-anti Beta 2 glycoprotein I antibodies are associated with clinical manifestations of the antiphosphoplipid syndrome. ACR/ARHP Scientific meeting 2009, Philadelphia.

Albers, G. W., Amarenco, P., Easton, J. D., Sacco, R. L., Teal, P., & American College of Chest Physicians (2008). Antithrombotic and thrombolytic therapy for ischemic stroke: American College of Chest Physicians Evidence-Based Clinical Practice Guidelines (8th Edition). *Chest*, *133*(6), 630S–669S.

Asherson, R. A. (2006). New subsets of the antiphospholipid syndrome. *Autoimmune Review*, *6*(2), 76–80.

Asherson, R. A., & Cervera, R. (2008). Microvascular and microangiopathic antiphospholipid-associated syndromes ("MAPS"): Semantic or antisemantic? *Autoimmunity Reviews*, *7*(3), 164–167.

Asherson, R. A., Cervera, R., de Groot, P. G., Erkan, D., Boffa, M.-C., Piette, J. C., Khamashta, M. A., & Shoenfeld, Y. (2003). Catastrophic antiphospholipid syndrome: International consensus statement on classification criteria and treatment guidelines. *Lupus*, *12*(7), 530–534.

Bates, S., Greer, I., Pabinger, I., Sofaer, S., & Hirsh, J. (2008). Venous Thromboembolism, Thrombophilia, Antithrombotic Therapy, and Pregnancy: American College of Chest Physicians Evidence-Based Clinical Practice Guidelines (8th Edition). *Chest*, *133*(6), 844S–886S.

Belilos, E., & Carson, S. (2009). Antiphospholipid syndrome. Medscape. Online at: http://emedicine.medscape.com/article/333221-overview (accessed August 2009).

Bermas, B., Erkan, D., & Shur, P. (2010). Diagnosis of the antiphospholipid syndrome. UpToDate, Last literature review version 18.3: September 2010. This topic last updated February 13, 2010.

Bertolaccini, M. L., Gomez, S., Pareja, J. F., Theodoridou, A., Sanna, G., et al. (2005). Antiphospholipid antibody tests: Spreading the net. *Annals of the Rheumatic Diseases*, *64*(11), 1639–1643.

Branch, D. W., Silver, R. M., Blackwell, J. L., Reading, J. C., & Scott, J. R. (1992). Outcome of treated pregnancies in women with antiphospholipid syndrome: An update of the Utah experience. *Obstetrics & Gynecology*, *80*(4), 614–620.

Buller, H. R., Agnelli, G., Hull, R. D., Hyers, T. M., Prins, M. H., & Raskob, G. E. (2004). Antithrombotic therapy for venous thromboembolic disease: The Seventh ACCP Conference on Antithrombotic and Thrombolytic Therapy. *Chest*, *126*, 401S–428S.

Bumas, B., & Schur, P. (2010). Pathogenesis of the antiphospholipid syndrome. UpToDate, Last literature review version 18.3: September 2010, updated: February 13, 2010.

Campbell, A. L., Pierangeli, S. S., Wellhausen, S., & Harris, E. N. (1995). Comparison of the effects of anticardiolipin antibodies from patients with the antiphospholipid syndrome and with syphilis on platelet activation and aggregation. *Thrombosis and Haemostasis*, *73*(3), 529–534.

Cervera, R., & Asherson, R. A. (2003). Clinical and epidemiological aspects in the antiphospholipid syndrome. *Immunobiology*, *207*(1), 5–11.

Cervera, R., Piette, J.-C., Khamashta, M. A., Shoenfeld, Y., & Camps, M. T. (2002). Antiphospholipid syndrome: Clinical and immuno-logical manifestations and patterns of disease expression in a cohort of 1000 patients. *Arthritis Rheumatology*, *46*(4), 1019–1027.

Crowther, M. A., & Wisloff, F. (2005). Evidence based treatment of the antiphospholipid syndrome. II. Optimal anticoagulant ther-apy for thrombosis. *Thrombosis Research*, *115*(1–2), 3–8.

Cuadrado, M. J., Mujic, F., Monoz, E., Khamashta, M. A., & Hughes, G. R. (1997). Thrombocytopenia in the antiphospholipid syn-drome. *Annals of Rhematic Diseases*, *56*(3), 194–196.

Derksen, R., & de Groot, P. G. (2004). Clinical consequences of antiphospholipid antibodies. *The Netherlands Journal of Medicine*, *62*(8), 273–278.

Derksen, R., de Groot, P., & Kappelle, L. (2003). Low dose aspirin after ischemic stroke associated with antiphospholipid syn-drome. *Neurology*, *61*(1), 111–114.

Derksen, R., de Groot, P. G., Neiuwenhuis, H., & Christiaens, G. (2001). How to treat women with antiphospholipid antibodies in pregnancy? *Annals of the Rheumatic Diseases*, *60*(1), 1–3.

Erkan, D., & Lockshin, M. D. (2004). What is antiphospholipid syn-drome? *Current Rheumatolgy Reports*, *6*(6), 451–457.

Finazzi, G. (1997). The Italian registry of antiphospholipid antibod-ies. *Haematologica*, *82*(1), 101–105.

Finazzi, G., Marchioli, R., Brancaccio, V., Schinco, P., Wisloff, F., et al. (2005). A randomized clinical trial of high-intensity warfarin vs. conventional antithrombotic therapy for the prevention of recur-rent thrombosis in patients with the antiphospholipid syndrome. *Journal of Thrombosis and Haemostasis*, *3*(5), 848–853.

Giannakopoulos, B., Passam, F., Ioannou, Y., & Krilis, S. A. (2009). How we diagnose the antiphospholipid syndrome. *Blood*, *113*(5), 985–994.

Girardi, G., Lockshin, M., & Salmon, J. (2007). The Antiphos-pholipid syndrome as a disorder initiated by inflammation:

Implications for the therapy of pregnant patients. *Nature Clinical Practice Rheumatology*, *3*(3), 140–147.

Gorki, H., Malinovski, V., & Stanbridge, R. D. (2008). The antiphospholipid syndrome and heart valve surgery. *European Journal of Cardiothoracic Surgery*, *33*(2), 168–181.

Hawkins, C., Gatenby, P., Tuck, R., Danta, G., & Andrews C. (2006). Cerebrovascular disease associated with antiphospholipid antibodies: More questions than answers. *Journal of Autoimmune Diseases*, *3*(3), doi:10.1186/1740-2557-3-3

Hedge, V. A. P., Vivas, Y., Shah, H., Hayborn, D., Srinivasan, V., & Gradman, A. (2007). Cardiovascular surgery outcomes in patients with the antiphospholipid syndrome — a case series. *Heart, Lung and Circulation*, *16*(6), 423–427.

Hirsh, J., Guyatt, G., Albers, G. W., Harrington, R., & Schünemann, H. (2008). Antithrombotic and thrombolytic therapy: American College of Chest Physicians Evidence-Based Clinical Practice Guidelines (8th Edition). *Chest*, *133*, 110S–112S.

Hughes, G. (1983). Thrombosis, abortion, cerebral disease, and the lupus anticoagulant. *British Medical Journal*, *287*(6399), 1088–1089.

Hughes, G., & Khamashta, M. (2003). Seronegative antiphospholipid syndrome. *Annals of the Rheumatic Diseases*, *62*(12), 1127.

Koniari, I., Siminelakis, S., Baikoussis, N., Papadopoulos, G., Goudevenos, J., & Apostolakis, E. (2010). Antiphospholipid syndrome; its implications in cardiovascular disease: A review. *Journal of Cardiovascular Surgery*, *5*, 101.

Levine, S. R., Brey, R. L., Tilley, B. C., Thompson, J. L., Sacco, R. L., et al. (2004). Antiphospholipid antibodies and subsequent thrombo-occlusive events in patients with ischemic stroke. *Journal of the American Medical Association*, *291*(5), 576–584.

Levine S., Deegan, M., Futrell, N., & Welch, K. (1990). Cerebrovascular and neurologic disease associated with antiphospholipid antibodies: 48 cases. *Neurology*, *40*(8), 1181–1189.

Lim, W. (2009). Antiphospholipid antibody syndrome. *Hematology*, *233*, 233–239.

Lima, F., Khamashta, M. A., Buchanan, N. M., Kerslake, S., Hunt, B. J., & Hughes, G. R. (1996). A study of sixty pregnancies in patients with the antiphospholipid syndrome. *Clinical and Experimental Rheumatology*, *14*(2), 131–136.

Lynch, A., Marlar, R., Murphy, J., Davila, G., Santos, M., et al. (1994). Antiphospholipid antibodies in predicting adverse pregnancy outcome. A prospective study. *Annals of Intern Medicine, 120,* 470–475.

McNeil, H. P., Chesterman, C. N., & Krilis, S. A. (1991). Immunology and clinical importance of antiphospholipid antibodies. *Advances in Immunology, 49,* 193–280.

Merrill, J. T., Shen, C., Gugnani, M., Lahita, R. G., & Mongey, A. B. (1997). High prevalence of antiphospholipid antibodies in patients taking procainamide. *Journal of Rheumatology, 24*(6), 1083–1088.

Miyakis, S., Lockshin, M. D., Atsumi, T., Branch, D. W., Brey, R., et al. (2006). International consensus statement on an update of the classification criteria for definite antiphospholipid syndrome (APS). *Journal of Thrombosis and Haemostasis, 4*(2), 295–306.

Ortel, T. (2005). Thrombosis and the antiphospholipid syndrome. *Hematology (American Society of Hematology Education Program),* 462–468.

Out, H. J., Kooijman, C. D., Bruinse, H. W., Derksen, R. (1991). Histopathological findings in placentae from patients with intra-uterine fetal death and antiphospholipid antibodies. *European Journal of Obstetrics & Gynecology and Reproductive Biology, 41*(3), 179–186.

Pengo, V., Graffiti, A., Legman, C., Gresele, P., Barcellona, D., et al. (2010). Clinical course of high-risk patients diagnosed with antiphospholipid syndrome. *Journal of Thrombosis and Haemostasis, 8*(2), 237–242.

Pengo, V., Tripod, A., Reber, G., Rand, J. H., Ortel, T. L., et al. (2009). Update of the guidelines for lupus anticoagulant detection. Subcommittee on Lupus Anticoagulant/Antiphospholipid Antibody of the Scientific and Standardization Committee of the International Society on Thrombosis and Haemostasis. *Journal of Thrombosis and Haemostasis, 7*(10), 1737–1740.

Roubey, R. A. (1994). Autoantibodies to phospholipid-binding plasma proteins: A new view of lupus anticoagulants and other "antiphospholipid" autoantibodies. *Blood, 84*(9), 2854–2867.

Ruffatti, A., Ross, T. D., Ciprian, M., Bertero, M. T., Salvatore, S., et al. (2011). Risk factors for a first thrombotic event in antiphospholipid antibody carriers: A prospective multicentre follow-up study. *Annals of the Rheumatic Diseases, 2011* (Feb 1). [Epub ahead of print]

Ruiz-Irastorza, G., & Khamashta, M. A. (2005). Stroke and antiphospholipid syndrome: The treatment debate. *Rheumatology, 44*(8), 971–974.

The Stroke Prevention in Reversible Ischemia Trial (SPIRIT) Study Group (1997). A randomized trial of anticoagulants versus aspirin after cerebral ischemia of presumed arterial origin. *Annals of Neurology, 42*(6), 857–865.

Tsagalis, G., Psimenou, N., & Laggouranis, A. (2010). Effective treatment of antiphospholipid syndrome with plasmapheresis and rituximab. *Hippokratia, 14*(3), 215–216.

Weiss, S., Nyzio, J. B., Cines, D., Detre, J., Milas, B. L., et al. (2008). Antiphospholipid syndrome: Intraoperative and postoperative anticoagulation in cardiac surgery. *Journal of Cardiothoracic Vascular Anesthesia, 22*(5), 735–739.

Wilson, W. A., Gharavi, A. E., Koike, T., Lockshin, M. D., Branch, D. W., et al. (1999). International consensus statement on preliminary classification criteria for definite antiphospholipid syndrome. *Arthritis and Rheumatism, 42*(7), 1309–1311.

Vasculitis of the Central Nervous System and Cranial Vessel (Arteritis)

Alice E. Davis

Evidence-Based Nursing Care for Stroke and Neurovascular Conditions,
First Edition. Edited by Sheila A. Alexander.
© 2013 John Wiley & Sons, Inc. Published 2013 by John Wiley & Sons, Inc.

HISTORICAL PERSPECTIVE

Numerous names have been assigned to giant cell (temporal) arteritis (GCA) based on the historical recounts or the histological features of the disease. GCA was first attributed to Hutchinson in 1890, who described inflamed temporal arteries on an elderly man who was unable to wear his hat. Later, in 1932, Horton linked clinical and histological features of the disease named after him (Horton's Disease). Histologically, giant cells, which are transformed macrophages characteristic of granulomatous lesions, have been identified in GCA. Consequently, terms such as giant cell arteritis and granulomatous arteritis have been used. Because it is a disease of those over 50 years of age, it has also been called arteritis of the aged (Kawasaki & Purvin, 2009).

DEFINITION AND CLASSIFICATION

GCA is a chronic, systemic, granulomatous vasculitis of large and medium vessels. It most often involves the cranial branches of the arteries originating from the aortic arch. These arteries divide at the neck and supply the head and temporal areas. Although these arteries are primarily involved, GCA can be widespread and involve other organ systems including the abdominal and thoracic aorta, extremities, and even the small bowel (Klein, Hunder, Stanson, & Sheps 1975; Evans, Bowles, Bjornsson, Mullany & Hunder, 1994; Annamalai, Francis, Ranatunga, & Resch, 2007).

In 1990, the American College of Rheumatology provided criteria for the classification of GCA (Hunder, Bloch, Michel, Stevens, Arend, & Calabrese, 1990) that continue to be used today (Table 13.1). The criteria were originally developed for research purposes and may not address variant forms of GCA including the occult GCA. When using the criteria, GSA is diagnosed if three out of five conditions are present, yielding a sensitivity of 93.5% and a specificity of 91.2% (Rahman & Rahman, 2005; Kawasaki & Purvin, 2009).

EPIDEMIOLOGY AND PATHOGENESIS

GCA is the most common form of primary vasculitis of adults in the Western world. Development of the disease is associated with distinctive age, ethnic, genetic, and inflammatory characteristics.

Table 13.1 The American College of Rheumatology 1990 criteria for the classification of giant cell arteritis

Age	Symptom development or findings in persons age 50 or older
Headache	New onset of headache or localized head pain
Abnormality of temporal artery	Tenderness with palpation, decreased pulsation, unrelated ateriosclerosis of cervical arteries
Elevated Erythrocyte sedimentation rate (ESR)	ESR ≥50 mm/hour
Artery Biopsy Abnormal	Artery biopsy characteristic of mononuclear cell infiltration or granulomatous inflammation, usually with multinucleated giant cells

Created from data in: Hunder, G.G., Bloch, D. A., Michel, B. A., Stevens, M. B., Arend, W. P., Calabrese L. H., et al. (1990). The American College of Rheumatology 1990 criteria for the classification of giant cell arteritis. *Arthritis & Rheumatism, 33*, 1122–1128.

There is an increased susceptibility for the disease distributed geographically in northern latitudes (Weyand & Goronzy, 2003). Persons of northern European decent are most at risk, with lowest rates found in persons of African, Asian, and Arab populations. However, others report a rise in GCA and polymyalgia rheumatica (PMR) incident rates in African Americans and Hispanic populations (Gonzalez, Varner, Lissie, Daniels, & Hokanson, 1989; Lam, Wirthlin, Gonzalez, Dubovy, & Feuer, 2007). GCA is a disease of persons over the age of 50, with a mean age of onset around 75 years. There is a preponderance of women diagnosed with the disease compared to men and often these women have a smoking history (Hunder, 2002; Salavarani, Crowson, O'Fallon, Hunder & Gabriel, 2004; Miller, 2007). There is a familial tendency, with clustering noted in family units. Cyclic variations have also been noted, with GCA with peak incident rates between 5 and 7 years, suggesting a trigger event or an infectious element may be causal factors of the disease (Salvarani, Gabriel, O'Fallon, & Hunder, 1995).

As a polygenetic disorder, GCA susceptibility has been reported along the human leukocyte antigen (HLA) regions of classes I and II, specifically HLA DRB1∗04 (Weyand, Hicok, Hunder, & Goronzy 1992; Gonzalez-Gay et al., 2007). There is also evidence that genes related to cytokine and chemokine can modulate the clinical expression of GCA potentially through polymorphism at the tumor necrosis factor-alpha locus and the interleukin (IL)-10 promotor region (Rueda, Roibas, Martin, & Gonzalez-Gay, 2007; Salvarani et al., 2007).

GCA has been linked to PMR through HLA-DR4. Interestingly, persons with PMR share a similar polymorphism sequence, suggesting it is pathogenetically related to GCA. PMR, also an inflammatory disorder, causes muscle pain and stiffness throughout the body, with pain most characteristically associated with muscles of the neck, shoulders, hips, and thighs. Although PMR is more common than GCA, there is evidence to support the theory that the conditions are two different expressions of the same vasculitic disorder. The pattern of T-cell–derived cytokines differentiates the two patient populations. Not only are these disorders linked, but 50% of patients with GCA develop PMR and up to 30% of patients with PMR develop GCA (Nordborg & Nordborg, 2004; Gonzalez-Gay, 2009). Features of the diseases are presented in Table 13.2. Other genetic associations are also speculated, especially those related to ischemic anterior optic neuropathy (IAON) (Weyand, Hicok, Hunder, & Goronzy, 1992; Hunder, 2010c).

PATHOPHYSIOLOGY

Although the exact cause of GCA is unknown, the clinical and laboratory features of GCA suggest an ongoing inflammatory process that likely targets the advential layer of the vessel and initiates the immune response. Both the cellular immune (t-lymphocytes) and humoral (antibody) systems are activated, perhaps by a viral infection. The systemic inflammatory response seems to predominate, causing an acute-phase response that results in inflammatory infiltrates of affected vessels. Along with lymphocytes and macrophages, giant cells of the Langerhans and foreign debris (likely vessel lining) are found. The lymphocytes are mostly of the CD4 positive cell type, with some CD8 cell types mentioned. The production of cytokines, most specifically interleukin-6 (IL-6), is also notable and seems to mediate the intensity of the response, as seen through the rise in acute phase proteins such as CRP, serum amyloid, A haptoglobin, fibrinogen, and complement. In addition, the Il-6 expression accounts for the clinical features of fever, anorexia, myalgias, and weight loss. Production of Il-6 also

Table 13.2 Features of Giant Cell Arteritis (GCA) and Polymyalgia Rhumatica (PMR)

Factors, Signs, Symptoms	GCA	PMR
Age at onset	50	50
Sex	Female /Male 3-4/1	Female /Male 3/1
Site of Inflammation		
Constitutional Signs/Symptoms	Fever Weight loss Fatigue	Fever Weight loss Fatigue
Symptoms	Headaches	Stiffness and aching neck, shoulders and hips (pelvic)
	Temporal headaches	
	Scalp pain along temporal artery	Swelling and stiffness in knees, hands, wrists, and ankles (synovial structures)
	Jaw claudication	
	Jaw weakness when chewing or talking	
	Weakness or pain in arm	
	Visual disturbances (diplopia, unilateral loss)	
	Internal organ involvement	
	Upper respiratory (cough, new sore throat)	
Laboratory	Elevated ESR , CRP, platelet count	Elevated ESR and CRP Normocytic anemia
Histology	Presence of granulomatous infiltrates w macrophages and CD4+ T cells in arterial wall; giant cells may not be present	Presence of mild synovitis w macrophages and CD4+ T cells

ESR erythrocyte sedimentation rate; CRP C-reactive Protein.
Created from data in Cantini, F., Niccoli, L., Nannini, C., Bertoni, M., & Salvarani (2008); Hunder, G. (2010a).

correlates with the severity and duration of the GCA symptoms rising and falling in response to glucocorticoid therapy (Goronzy & Weyand, 2002; Weyand & Goronzy, 2003). The second or humoral response represents a maladaptive antigen-specific response probably from antigen presenting dendritic cells that attack the vessel wall, causing the ischemic changes seen in GCA (Kawasaki

& Purvin, 2009). Consequences of the inflammatory process are patchy infiltrations of both small and large arterial vessels (branches of the external carotid arteries, thoracic aorta, cervical arteries), thrombosis, and vessel occlusion or stricture. Damage to the smooth muscle of the media further increases scarring, fibrosis, and narrowing and may be accompanied by a systemic inflammatory response. Further, it is hypothesized that certain cytokine expression may be linked to the clinical expression of GCA. For example, persons with higher levels of interleukin-2 had symptoms of PMR while persons with ischemic artery involvement had higher levels of interferon gamma and interleukin-1beta mRNA (Weyand et al., 1997).

DIAGNOSTIC APPROACH
History
The clinical onset of GCA may be gradual occurring over many months, but in some patients there is an acute onset of symptoms. Because the vasculitis can involve many systems, the history must be used to probe for symptoms in the cardiovascular, respiratory, neurological, and integumentary systems in addition to symptoms related to the eye. History of PMR should indicate a high risk for GCA and prompt further questions related to musculoskeletal system involvement. Table 13.3 outlines the clinical features associated with GCA and guides the approach to history and physical examination.

Physical examination features
Individuals affected with GCA appear chronically ill and present with constitutional signs such as fever, anorexia, and weight loss. Prominent frontal or parietal branches of the temporal artery may be tender, nodular, or thickened, with absent or decreased pulsation of the artery. These findings of tenderness and prominence are less often appreciated in the occipital, post-auricular, or facial arteries. Scalp tenderness, usually in the temporal area, with complaints of a "pin-pricking" sensation occurs and may be accompanied by a headache. Scalp ischemia or necrosis may be present, especially in the temporal-parietal regions.

Because of vascular inflammation, other body systems are also at risk for the development of GCA. Therefore, a thorough

Table 13.3 Clinical Manifestations of GCA

Pain	**Neurological**
Jaw Claudication	Stroke
Temporal artery pain or abnormality	Ischemia (vertebral and carotid arteries)
Scalp tenderness	Dementia
Generalized headache	Psychosis
Temporal headache	Coma
	Subarachnoid hemorrhage
Vision	Neuropathies (various peripheral types)
Diplopia	
Vision loss (unilateral-bilateral)	**Systemic features of inflammation**
Monocular blindness	Anorexia
Amaurosis	Asthenia
AION	Malaise
Retinal artery occlusion	Myalgia
Horner's pupil	Arthralgia
Efferent pupil abnormalities	Weight Loss
	Fever
Audiovestibular	
Hearing loss	**Cardiovascular**
Vertigo	Athrosclerosis
Disequilibrium	Plaque destabilization
Dizziness	Angina
Tinnitus	Aortic aneurysms
Oral	**Other**
Odontogenic pain	Small bowel infarction
Trismus	Kidney, lung, heart involvement
Throat pain	Occult Features
Tongue or lip infarction	

AION: Anterior ischemic optic neuropathy or ateritic AION. Adapted from: Cantini, et al. (2008).

physical examination should involve the monitoring of the following systems.

Cardiovascular system

Check for diminished pulses, blood pressure differences, abdominal bruits, and other pulse discrepancies. Temporal arteries should be examined for tenderness, erythema, nodules, or swelling.

Respiratory system

Symptoms may be mild or absent but may include cough or upper respiratory tract symptoms.

Neurological system

Check for evidence of transient ischemic attacks, subacute stroke findings, transient or fixed visual changes, diplopia, ocular motor weakness, pale swollen optic disc, difficulty swallowing, or tongue infarction. Vertigo, hearing loss, and carotid artery lesions may also be present.

Integumentary system

Check for scalp tenderness, ischemia, or head or skin lesions.

Musculoskeletal system

Check for pain and stiffness in neck, shoulders, hips, and thighs. Check for jaw claudication and differentiate from temporal mandibular joint disorder (for jaw claudication, pain ceases with resting of the muscle). Snovitis or distal extremity swelling and arm claudication can be found.

DIAGNOSIS

There is no single diagnostic examination, sign, or symptom that assures the diagnosis of GCA syndrome. There are often inconsistencies in patient presentations and patients present with various combinations of clinical and diagnostic features. Diagnosis is based on clinical features, and a high index of suspicion for GCA can often trump a negative biopsy. However, a dual approach to diagnosis using the cluster of characteristic symptoms/signs and biopsy evidence of inflammation and vasculopathy has lead to successful treatment. Therefore, the optimal workup for diagnosing GCA includes history, clinical presentation, temporal artery biopsy, laboratory tests, and imaging studies. There are several differential diagnoses to consider when working up a patient for GCA, which include, but are not limited to, primary systemic amyloidosis, Takayasu's arteritis, and isolated angitis of the central nervous system (Cantini et al., 2008).

CLINICAL FEATURES

Although the diagnostic criteria for GCA propose classic clinical features including sudden onset of a headache, temporal artery tenderness on palpation, pulseless artery, or transient visual loss, the inflammatory component of GCS makes systemic features highly

Table 13.4 Onset Patterns of Clinical and Subclinical Variants of GCA

Type	Pattern
Typical GCA	Gradual onset in female > 70 years, fronto-temporal headache, jaw claudication, scalp tenderness, fever, and other constitutional symptoms
Typical GCA with PMR	Typical onset of GCA symptoms but are often overlooked due to pain and functional loss of hips and lower extremities. Occurs in 50% of patients.
GCA with normal ESR	High suscipician of GCA with normal ESR. High risk of vision loss with no systemic manifestations, elevated platelet levels and low ESR and CRP.
PMR with silent GCA	Later development of GCA in patients with PMR. If systemic symptoms arise, need temporal artery biopsy.
Fever of unknown origin	High risk of GCA in older persons with fever of unknown origin. May need to consider temporal artery biopsy once other disease are excluded.
Vision loss with occult GCA	Vision loss may be a first manifestation of silent GCA; older patients with visual disturbances should be evaluated for acute phase reactant and started on steroids.
Isolated extracranial large vessel GCA	Suspect large-vessel GCA in older persons with chest pain radiating to the interscapular area or with ischemic features of the upper extremities.

Adapted from Cantini et al. (2008).

likely. In Table 13.2 clinical features related to numerous body systems are outlined.

In addition to cranial arteritis, two other clinical subtypes have been described. These include systemic inflammatory syndrome and large vessel vasculitis (Kawaskai & Purvin, 2009). Cantini et al. (2008) provide a further breakdown of clinical types and patterns of onset (Table 13.4) that must be considered in the diagnosis of GCA.

DIAGNOSTIC TESTING
Laboratory
C-reactive protein (CRP)
CRP – a marker of inflammation – has a rapid response time for inflammation and has little sensitivity to age, gender, or blood factors. A high sensitivity (98%) in GCA has been reported (Hayreh,

Podhajsky, Raman, & Zimmerman, 1997; Gonzalex-Gay et al., 2005; Parikh et al., 2006).

Erythrocyte sedimentation rate (ESR)

ESR is a measure of body inflammation. An ESR higher than 50 mm/hr alone is not diagnostic of GCA. If GCA is suspected, an elevated ESR can support the diagnosis, but conversely a low or normal ESR does not rule out GCA. ESR levels are elevated by multiple factors including infection, inflammation, connective tissue disorders, malignancy, hypercholesterolanemia, trauma, as well as age and female gender. Many patients with GCA may have continued low ESR if they have concomitant conditions such as heart failure, impaired protein synthesis, or take anti-inflammatory medications. The availability of the ESR makes it a useful diagnostic test for GCA despite its lack of sensitivity and specificity. There is some speculation that an acute phase response, which includes fever, weight loss, anemia, and an ESR higher than 85 mm/hr, indicates a low risk of cerebral ischemic injury (Hayreh, Podhajsky, Raman, & Zimmerman, 1997). There is also speculation that a strong initial anti-inflammatory response associated with the need for high-dose steroids heralds a longer duration of therapy (Herdandez-Rodriquez et al., 2002). However, neither of these relationships has been supported by others.

Thrombocytosis

An elevated platelet count or thrombocytosis (increased platelets higher than $375,000/mm^3$), along with an elevated ESR, may be helpful for ruling in GCA (Foroozan et al., 2002). Many patients with constitutional symptoms of GCA also presented with a positive GCA biopsy, elevated ESR, and increased CRP (Gonzalex-Gay et al., 2005).

Temporal artery biopsy (TAB)

TAB is considered the gold standard for diagnosing GCA, but it is not without limitations. A histological feature of the temporal artery is granulomatous inflammation. Diagnosis by biopsy is not without challenges; the specimen may consist of patchy, not consistent, granulomatous inflammation, or changes may not be seen if the length of the specimen is not sufficient. Bilateral biopsies may be necessary to improve diagnostic yield (Belliveau & ten Hove, 2011). Even with an optimal biopsy technique, false negatives occur in greater than 9% of cases (Hunder, 2010b).

Imaging studies

There has been some support for the use of ultrasonograpy (US) as a means to diagnose the "halo sign" that occurs as a result of temporal artery edema. Sensitivity and specificity of the sign with acceptable technical quality were comparable to other rheumatology related autoantibody diagnostic tests, and recommendations have been made to add US to the diagnostic criteria (Arida, Kyprianou, Kanakis, & Sfikakis, 2010). If extracranial GCA is suspected, angiography, CT scan, and MRI should be considered in an effort to reveal inflammatory changes, even though their diagnostic accuracy has not been defined.

TREATMENT

Glucocorticoid therapy is the treatment for GCA and should be initiated without delay if the diagnosis of GCA is strongly suspected. Often, there is no biopsy evidence of arteritis even in the face of strong clinical suspicion. Although glucocorticoid administration has never been tested in placebo-controlled trials, use of glucocorticoids for GCA is well established and has been deemed safe and efficacious (Hunder, 2010b). With that being said, the challenge of treating an elderly population with numerous co-morbidities cannot be underestimated. Therefore, the goal of therapy must focus on suppression of the inflammation while limiting the complications associated with GCA and the co-morbidities common in this age group, such as diabetes, heart disease, heart failure, hypertension, and osteoporosis (Cantini, Niccoli, Nannini, Bertoni, & Salvarani, 2008).

While there is no consensus on the type, route, or duration of corticosteroid therapy, oral dosing with prednisone seems to be the preferred method of steroid administration. However, there have been some reports that pulse dosing with intravenous methylprednisolone may have greater benefits than oral dosing with prednisone, but these trials are small and as of yet unconfirmed (Mazlumzadeh et al., 2006; Hunder, 2010). Initial dosing with prednisone is not exact but ranges between 40 mg and 60 mg daily in single or divided doses. The therapeutic aim is to rapidly reduce symptoms and limit incidence of ocular complications. Once administered, therapy should be continued to rapidly alleviate relieve or reduce the symptoms. Smaller doses as low as 20 mg daily have been reported as efficacious, but there is the possibility of undertreatment with this lower dose and therefore it is not often used (Hunder, 2011b).

Corticosteroid tapering

The course of treatment for GCA is long and may extend over a period of 1 to 2 years. Two end points are pivotal in the decision to taper corticoid doses: remission of symptoms and normalization of inflammatory markers (ESR and CRP). Tapering recommendations focus on individual patient response to therapy and clinical judgment of the provider. However, there is support for maintaining the initial dose for 2–4 weeks followed by a 10% reduction of the total daily dose until 10 mg/day is reached, which should be followed by a gradual decrease in dose by 1–2 mg every month until therapy is completed (Cantini et al., 2008; Hunder, 2010b).

Treatment in the presence of visual loss

There is strong support for the rapid administration of high-dose glucocorticoids in the presence of new onset visual loss. Time to initiation of therapy was a predictor for blindness (Nordborg & Nordborg, 2004), and treatment initiated within 24 hours of symptom onset improved visual symptoms in 57% of patients (Gonzalez-Gay, Blanco et al., 1998). Rapid treatment can prevent visual loss but unfortunately there are no studies that support recovery of fixed visual loss once it has occurred. Predictors and responses to treatment vary based on clinical manifestations. Patients with transient visual loss and jaw claudication were at higher risk for permanent visual loss, and cerebrovascular events were more likely to occur in patients with permanent vision loss and/or jaw claudication. These risks are described even in the presence of corticosteroid therapy. There was a decrease in risk of developing permanent visual loss if constitutional signs or elevated liver enzymes were present (Gonzalez-Gay et al., 1998).

Other therapies

Antiplatelet therapy, specifically low-dose aspirin 81–100 mg/day, is recommended for all GCA patients. The recommendation is supported by two retrospective studies that found a reduction in risk for visual loss and cerebral ischemic events in patients with GCA who were taking aspirin for cardiovascular disease prior to GCA onset (Nesher et al., 2004; Lee, Smith, Galor, & Hoffman, 2006). Other consideration in the use of aspirin is the risk of visual loss in GCA patients. Aspirin may be useful in reducing thrombotic risk associated with narrowed lumens of the posterior ciliary and ophthalmic arteries and reduce risk of vision loss in patients with thrombocytosis (platelet counts higher than 400,000).

Methotrexate as a glucocorticoid-sparing strategy has met with mixed reviews in two randomized control trials (Jover et al., 2001; Hoffman et al., 2002). Treatment with methotrexate as a steroid-sparing agent in GCA is moderate and therefore the routine use of methotrexate in GCA is not recommended unless the individual is at high risk for adverse effects from prednisone.

Granulomatous inflammation is a key feature of GCA, suggesting that the use of a tissue necrosis factor (TNF) inhibitor would be a beneficial treatment. In a controlled randomized trial, infliximab, a TNF alpha inhibitor, did not reduce the number of patients with relapse and did not increase the number of patients for whom tapering off prednisone avoided relapse (Hoffman et al., 2007).

Follow-Up

Especially challenging during corticosteroid tapering is gauging disease activity. Both recurrent disease and flares in GCA are problematic when tapering corticosteroids. Flares do not typically occur when prednisone doses are higher than 15mg/day, but flares occur more often at lower doses. Although imperfect biomarkers of disease, acute phase reactants such as ESR and CRP should be monitored throughout the treatment phase and more closely if flares or relapse are suspected. Il-6 and soluble intercellular adhesion molecules are promising assays for assessing active disease, and relapse was more closely associated with elevations in IL-6 than with ERS (Weyand, Fulbright, Hunder, Evans, & Goronzy, 2000).

Relapse

Relapse must be considered under three circumstances: (1) return of symptoms similar to those from the initial presentation; (2) new symptoms of GCA or PMR occur; or (3) acute phase reactants (ESR or CRP) elevate. Treatment may be prolonged if relapses require treatment with corticosteroids (Hunder, 2010b). Patient should receive close follow-up if reoccurrences or relapse is suspected.

Complications

The need to use glucocorticoids for prolonged periods of time in GCA is problematic. In addition to weight gain, hypertension, and opportunistic infection, there is also the threat of developing glucose intolerance and diabetes mellitus. Long-term use may lead to or exacerbate osteoporosis. Adjunctive treatment when using glucocorticoids should include calcium and vitamin D supplements and monitoring of bone mineral density at the onset and duration of treatment. Hormone replacement and bisphosphonates should also be considered (Hunder, 2010b).

Large-vessel vasculitis may occur as a primary feature of GCA or may develop as a later complication of the disease (Kawasaki & Prvin, 2009). Subclinical aortitis found in over 50% of GCA patients is being considered a prominent feature of the disease rather than a complication. Aortic aneurysm or dissection is estimated to occur in one out of five patients with GCA (Nuenninghoff & Matteson, 2003). Risk factors for the development of aortic aneurysm in GCA patients includes: aortic insufficiency murmur, PMR diagnosis, and ERS higher than 100 mm/hr, or a combination of any two of the following problems: PMR, hyperlipidemia, hypertension, and coronary artery disease (Bongartz & Matteson, 2006). Clearly those patients who have a high-risk profile for developing aneurysms should undergo routine screening in order to detect early changes. Screening strategies should include as a minimum an abdominal ultrasound, chest X-ray, and transthoracic echocardiogram yearly (Bongartz & Matteson, 2006). Patients presenting with chest pain, radiating to the interscapular area or with symptoms of reduced blood supply to the upper extremities should be examined for arterial bruits and diminished radial and ulnar pulses especially if these symptoms are associated with an increase in acute phase reactants (Brack, Martinez-Taboada, Stanson, Goronzy, & Weyand, 1999).

PROGNOSIS

Interestingly, the natural history of GCA is spontaneous remission. However, the natural course of the disease may be prolonged for many years. Thus, without intervention, there is a high rate of morbidity related to the ischemic complication caused by the inflammatory process. Therefore, the aim is to recognized the disease early, reduce inflammation, and prevent ischemic complications that include blindness, neurological dysfunction, and infarction of other organs (Kawasaki and Purvin, 2009).

REFERENCES

Annamalai, A., Francis, M., Ranatunga, S., & Resch, D. (2007). Giant cell arteritis presenting as small bowel infarction. *Journal of General Internal Medicine*, *22*, 140–144.

Arida, A., Kyprianou, M., Kanakis, M., & Sfikakis, P. (2010). The diagnostic value of ultrasonography-derived edema of the temporal artery wall in giant cell arteritis: A second meta-analysis. *BMC Musculoskeletal Disorders*, *11*, 44.

Belliveau, M., & ten Hove, M. (2011). Five things to know about giant cell arteritis. *Canadian Medical Association Journal*, *183*(5), 581.

Bongartz, T., & Matteson, E. (2006). Large vessel involvement in giant cell arteritis. *Current Opinion in Rheumatology*, *18*, 10–17.

Brack, A., Martinez-Taboada, V., Stanson, A., Gononzy, J., & Weyand, C. (1999). Disease pattern in cranial and large-vessel giant cell arteritis. *Arthritis & Rheumatism*, *42*(2), 311–317.

Cantini, F., Niccoli, L., Nannini, C., Bertoni, M., & Salvarani C. (2008). Diagnosis and treatment of giant cell arteritis. *Drugs and Aging*, *25*(4), 281–297.

Evans, J., Bowles, C., Bjornsson, J., Mullany, C., & Hunder, G. (1994). Thoracic aortic aneurysm and rupture in giant cell arteritis. A descriptive study of 41 cases. *Arthritis & Rheumatism*, *37*(10), 1539–1547.

Foroozan, R., Danesh-Meyer, H., Salvino, P., Gamble, G., Mekan-Sabbagh, O., & Sergott, R. (2002). Thrombocytosis in patients with biopsy-proven giant cell arteritis. *Ophthalmology*, *109*, 1267–1271.

Gonzalez, E. B., Varner, W. T., Lissie, J. R., Daniels, J. C., & Hokanson, J. A. (1989). Giant-cell arteritis in the southern United States: An

11-year retrospective study from the Texas Gulf Coast. *Archives of Internal Medicine*, *149*(7), 1561–1565.

Gonzalez-Gay, M., Blanco, R., Rodriguez-Valverdere, V., Martinez-Taboada, V., Delgado-Rodriguez, M., et al. (1998). Permanent visual loss and cerebrovascular accidents in giant cell arteritis: Predictors and response to treatment. *Arthritis & Rheumatism*, *41*(8), 1497–1504.

Gonzalez-Gay, M. A., Lopez-Diaz, M. J., Barros, S., Garcia-Porrua, C., Sanchez-Andrade, A., et al. (2005). Giant cell arteritis: Laboratory tests at the time of diagnosis in a series of 240 patients. *Medicine*, *84*(5), 277–290.

Gonzalez-Gay, M. A., Rueda, B., Vilchez, J., Lopez-Nevot, M., Robledo, G., et al. (2007). Contribution of MHC class I region to genetic susceptibility for giant cell arteritis. *Rheumatology (Oxford)*, *46*(3), 431–434.

Goronzy, J., & Weyand, C. (2002). Cytokines in giant cell arteritis. *Cleveland Clinic Journal of Medicine*, *69*(Suppl. 2), 91–94.

Hayreh S. S., Podhajsky, P. A, Raman, R., & Zimmerman, B. (1997). Giant cell arteritis: Validity and reliability of various diagnostic criteria. *American Journal of Ophthalmology*, *123*, 285–296.

Hernández-Rodríguez, J., García-Martínez, A., Casademont, J., Filella, X., Esteban, M., et al. (2002). A strong initial systemic inflammatory response is associated with higher corticosteroid requirements and longer duration of therapy in patients with giant-cell arthritis. *Arthritis & Rheumatism*, *47*(1), 29–35.

Hoffman, C., Cid, M., Hellman, D., Stone, J., Schousboe, J., et al. (2002). A multicenter, randomized, double blind, placebo-controlled trial of adjuvant methotrexate treatment for giant cell arteritis. *Arthritis & Rheumatism*, *46*(5), 1309–1318.

Hoffman, G., Cid, M., Rendt-Zagar, K., Merkel, P., Weyand, C., et al. (2007). Infliximab-GCA Study Group. Infliximab for maintenance of glucocorticosteroid-induced remission of giant cell arteritis: A randomized trial. *Annals of Internal Medicine*, *146*(9), 621–630.

Hunder, G. (2002). Epidemiology of giant cell arteritis. *Cleveland Clinic Journal of Medicine*, *69* (Suppl. 2), 79–82.

Hunder, G. G. (2008). Pathogenesis of giant cell (temporal) arteritis. UpToDate. Last update June 28, 2008. Literature review current through July 2012.

Hunder, G. G. (2010a). Clinical manifestations of giant cell (temporal) arteritis. UpToDate. Last update November 29, 2011. Literature review current through July 2012.

Hunder, G. G. (2010b). Diagnosis of giant cell (temporal) arteritis. UpToDate. Last update September 29, 2008. Literature review current through July 2012.

Hunder, G. G. (2010c). Pathogenesis of giant cell (temporal) arteritis. UpToDate. Last update June 12, 2012. Literature review current through July 2012.

Hunder, G. G., Bloch, D. A., Michel, B. A., Stevens, M. B., Arend, W. P., et al. (1990). The American College of Rheumatology 1990 criteria for the classification of giant cell arteritis. *Arthritis & Rheumatism*, *33*, 1122–1128.

Jover, J., Hernandez-Garcia, C., Morado, I., Vargas, E., Banares, A. & Fernandez Gutierrez, B. (2001). Combined treatment of giant cell arteritis with methotrexate and prednisone. A randomized, double blind, placebo-controlled trial. *Annals of Internal Medicine*, *134*, 106–114.

Kawasaki, A., & Purvin, V. (2009). Giant cell arteritis: An updated review. *Acta Ophthalmologica*, *87*, 13–32.

Klein, R., Hunder, G., Stanson, A., & Sheps, S. (1975). Large artery involvement in giant cell (temporal) arteritis. *Annals of Internal Medicine*, *83*, 806–812.

Lam, B. L., Wirthlin, R. S., Gonzalez, A., Dubovy, S. R., & Feuer, W. J. (2007). Giant cell arteritis among Hispanic Americans. *American Journal of Ophthalmology*, *143*(1), 161–163.

Lee, M., Smith, S., Galor, A., & Hoffman, G. (2006). Antiplatelet and anticoagulant therapy in patients with giant cell arteritis. *Arthritis & Rheumatism*, *54*, 3306–3309.

Mazlumzadeh, M., Hunder, G., Easley, K., Calamia, K., Matteson, E., et al. (2006). Treatment of giant cell arteritis using induction therapy with high-dose glucocorticoids: A double-blind, placebo-controlled, randomized prospective clinical trial. *Arthritis & Rheumatism*, *54*, 3310–3318.

Miller, N. (2007). Epidemiology of giant cell arteritis on an Arab population: A 22-year study. *British Journal of Ophthalmology*, *91*, 705–706.

Nesher, G., Berkun, Y., Mates, M., Baras, M., Rubinow, A., & Sonnenblick, M. (2004). Low-dose aspirin and prevention of cranial ischemic complications in giant cell arteritis. *Arteritis & Rheumatism, 50*, 1332–1337.

Nuenninghoff, D., & Matteson, E. (2003). The role of disease modifying antirheumatic drugs in the treatment of giant cell arteritis. *Clinical and Experimental Rheumatology, 21*(Suppl. 32), 29–34.

Nordborg, E., & Nordborg, C. (2004). Giant cell arteritis: Strategies in diagnosis and treatment. *Current Opinion in Rheumatology, 16*, 25–30.

Parikh, M., Miller, N., Lee, A., Savino, P., Vacarezza, M., et al. (2006). Prevalence of a normal C-reactive protein with an elevated erythrocyte sedimentation rate in biopsy-proven giant cell arteritis. *Ophthalmology, 113*(10), 1842–1845.

Rahman, W., & Rahman, F. (2005). Giant cell (temporal) arteritis: An overview and update. *Survey Ophthalmology, 50*, 415–428.

Rueda, B., Roibas, B., Martin, J., & Gonzalez-Gay, M. (2007). Influence of interleukin 10 promoter polymorphisms in susceptibility to giant cell arteritis in Northwestern Spain. *Journal of Rheumatology, 34*(7), 1535–1539.

Salvarani, C., Casali, B., Farnetti, E., Pipitone, N., Formisano, D., et al. (2007). PlA1/A2 polymorphism of the platelet glycoprotein receptor IIIA and risk of cranial ischemic complications in giant cell arteritis. *Arthritis & Rheumatism, 56*(10), 3502–3508.

Salvarani, C., Crowson, C., O'Fallon, W., Hunder, G., & Gabriel, S. (2004). Reappraisal of the epidemiology of giant cell arteritis in Olstead County, Minnesota, over a fifty-year period. *Arthritis & Rheumatism, 51*, 264–268.

Salvarani, C., Gabriel, S., O'Fallon, W., & Hunder, G. (1995). The incidence of giant cell arteritis in Olmsted County, Minnesota: Apparent fluctuations in a cyclic pattern. *Annals of Internal Medicine, 123*(3), 192–194.

Weyand, C., Fulbright, J., Hunder, G., Evans, J., & Goronzy, J. (2000). Treatment of giant cell arteritis: Interleukin-6 as biologic marker of disease activity. *Arthritis & Rheumatism, 43*(5), 1041–1048.

Weyand, C. M., & Goronzy, J. J. (2003). Giant cell arteritis and polymyalgia rheumatica. *Annals of Internal Medicine, 139*, 505–515.

Weyand, C. M., Hicok, K. C., Hunder, G. G., & Goronzy, J. J. (1992). The HLA-DRB1 locus as a genetic component in giant cell arteritis. Mapping of a disease-linked sequence motif to the antigen-binding site of the HLA-DR molecule. *Journal of Clinical Investigation, 90*, 2355–2361.

Weyand, C. M., Tetzlaff, N., Björnsson, J., Brack, A., Younge, B., & Goronzy, J. J. (1997). Disease patterns and tissue cytokine profiles in giant cell arteritis. *Arthritis & Rheumatism, 40*(1), 19–26.

Index

Evidence-Based Nursing Care for Stroke and Neurovascular Conditions,
First Edition. Edited by Sheila A. Alexander.
© 2013 John Wiley & Sons, Inc. Published 2013 by John Wiley & Sons, Inc.